About the author

Margrit Coates was born with an extraordinary ability to tune into the needs of animals, particularly horses, but she suppressed her gifts for many years. Instead, she pursued a career in advertising and marketing, becoming the head of PR for a large company. She started riding in earnest in her mid-twenties and later through her work became very involved with British equestrian events. However, she always felt called to develop her healing abilities and therefore decided to retrain as a complementary practitioner and undertook a period of extensive study and exams. Word spread about her powerful healing ability and soon she established herself as an animal healer who specialises in treating horses. In addition to giving private consultations, lecturing and running courses on animal healing, she is the co-founder of Holistic Pets, a unique clinic offering natural treatments for animals.

The horse's healing prayer

Your hand has the power
To hurt me or to heal me,
Look into my eyes
To the heart of my soul
And choose to heal me.

        Margrit Coates

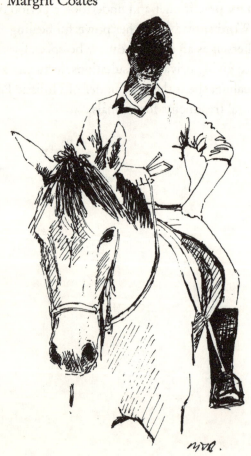

HEALING FOR HORSES

The Essential Guide to Using Hands-on Healing Energy with Horses

Margrit Coates

RIDER
LONDON · SYDNEY · AUCKLAND · JOHANNESBURG

I dedicate this book to Chocolate and Goldie
who gave me the best times of my life,
the sweetest memories. And to horses everywhere.

20 19

Published in 2001 by Rider, an imprint of Ebury Publishing

Ebury Publishing is a Random House Group company

Copyright © Margrit Coates 2001

Margrit Coates has asserted her right to be identified as the author of this Work in accordance with the Copyright, Designs and Patents Act 1988.

All rights reserved. No part of this publication may be reproduced, stored in a retrieval system, or transmitted in any form or by any means, electronic, mechanical, photocopying, recording or otherwise, without the prior permission of the copyright owner.

The Random House Group Limited Reg. No. 954009

Addresses for companies within the Random House Group can be found at www.randomhouse.co.uk

A CIP catalogue record for this book is available from the British Library

Penguin Random House is committed to a sustainable future for our business, our readers and our planet. This book is made from Forest Stewardship Council® certified paper.

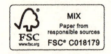

Printed and bound in Great Britain by Clays Ltd, Elcograf S.p.A.

Photography by Jon Banfield

ISBN 9780712601382

Copies are available at special rates for bulk orders. Contact the sales development team on 020 7840 8487 or visit www.booksforpromotions.co.uk for more information.

To buy books by your favourite authors and register for offers, visit www.randomhouse.co.uk

---

PLEASE NOTE:

Any information given in this book is not intended to be taken as a replacement for professional veterinary or medical advice. Hands-on healing is a complementary therapy to be used alongside the care, treatment and advice provided by a veterinary surgeon. A veterinary surgeon must always be consulted for any concerns or problems whatsoever with an equine. Neither the author nor the publisher can be held responsible for any loss or claim arising out of the use or misuse of the suggestions made in this book nor the failure to take professional veterinary advice. All information in this book is correct at the time of going to press to the best of the author's knowledge, but useful addresses etc may be subject to change, in which case they will be updated at the first opportunity.

Contents

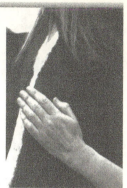

	Testimonials	vi
1	The path to the horse within	1
2	What is healing for horses?	18
3	Why horses need healing	39
4	Healing horses and the human link	65
5	Case histories	76
6	How to give a healing treatment	106
7	Healing for horses and chakras	131
8	Crystals and gemstones for healing	146
9	Other natural therapies	150
10	Using a healer for your horse	156
	Conclusion	160
	Useful addresses	162
	References and suggested further reading	164
	Author's acknowledgements	165
	Index	167

Testimonials

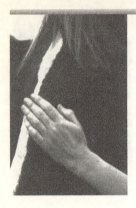

'To achieve the competitive edge in modern-day equestrian events, it is becoming increasingly necessary to maintain an open mind to all techniques that may enhance your horse's performance and wellbeing. To have a closed mind is to put oneself at a disadvantage.

'Although healing is not a new phenomenon, it is a sensitive subject that many of us have little understanding about. Margrit Coates is passionate about horses. Through this book, she has successfully tackled the difficult task of explaining healing in a way that most readers will easily comprehend.'

Blyth Tait MBE
Three Day Event Rider; Individual Gold Medal winner in Atlanta Olympic Games 1996; Olympic Bronze Medal winner Atlanta Games 1996 (with New Zealand team); World Champion 1990–1994, 1998–2002

'*Healing for Horses* is a book I thoroughly recommend every horse lover and veterinary surgeon to have on their bookshelves. The principles of healing are explained in a very "user friendly" way as well as being backed up by hard scientific fact. The beneficial and therapeutic effects of healing are well documented, with important emphasis being placed on preventative treatment and understanding the nature of the horse.

'This book is not just an interesting read, but an important manual for self-help therapy, which should result in a stronger human–equine bond.'

Cheryl Sears MVB, MRCVS, VETMFHOM
Homeopathic Veterinary Surgeon

'I heard of Margrit's skills through a professional colleague, who was unable to explain what she did, but was certain that "it worked" when all else failed. This coincided with a problem that I was grappling with at the time. Basher was suffering from a loss of performance that could not be explained by any conventional veterinary diagnostics. From being able to jump round a three-day event, he could now barely jump a three-foot show jump without knocking it down. The only abnormalities were noted when ridden: he found it difficult to bend through his neck to the left, and his right hind was weak, so that he tended to fall in to the right canter. Every effort had been made to coax the horse into jumping again, but to no avail, and he now seemed depressed and devoid of personality, presumably owing to a source of pain that I could not identify.

'Frustrated, my final strategy was to refer Basher to the equine oesteopath Anthony Pusey, with whom I had worked previously with much success. However, I thought that I would also trial Margrit's abilities on Basher. I accompanied Basher's owner to their first consultation and, without telling Margrit any of Basher's history, asked her what she thought his problem areas were. Over the course of an hour she pinpointed two areas of energy block, correlating exactly with the abnormalities under the saddle. I would make it clear that Margrit had not even seen the horse move, let alone ridden it: her entire consultation was conducted in a quiet stable. She also described how Basher had acquired such problems, detailing two falls in the previous two years that the owner had not realised were significant to the current problems.

'Astonishingly, Margrit talked about Basher's psychological state, affirming our concern that the horse was depressed. She then laid her hands on the horse and gave him healing. The owner, holding the horse, experienced the full effects of Basher's unhappiness and felt very emotionally moved. Basher went onto be successfully treated by Anthony Pusey, but osteopathy may not have been so effective without Margrit's prior healing treatment. The horse's personality quite definitely changed from the moment she treated him. From a clinical perspective I have been convinced of her insight and her accuracy on several occasions since.

'Margrit can point owners and veterinarians in the right direction, especially when conventional medicine fails. She seems able to visualise energy flow around a horse's body and thereby identify injury at sites of energy blockage. Her greatest skill lies in her understanding of the horse's psyche: she can communicate reassurance and positivity to a horse that has been mistreated or undiagnosed for too long. It is this that facilitates true healing.

'This is a book for anyone who wants to understand more about their horses.'

Major J. F. Holmes
MA Vet MB MRCVS RAVC
Regimental Veterinary Officer – Household Cavalry Mounted Regiment; regular contributor to *Horse* magazine

'I have used Margrit's healing for several of my horses and have found it invaluable to overcome some problems. In one particular case improvement was dramatic and immediate. I also find it fascinating to watch the healing treatments and see the horse's positive reaction to the energy work. I definitely feel that healing has a role to play in today's equestrian management. This book is a must for all horse lovers who wish to get the best out of their horses.'

Lucinda Fredericks
Champion Equestrian Sportswoman,
Australian Three Day Event Rider,
Grand Prix Dressage Rider

'I feel very privileged to have been allowed a glimpse of the contents of this book prior to publication. I had no preconceptions of what I would find or how I would feel, and certainly did not expect to be so profoundly captivated and moved by the contents.

'To my surprise, it took me back to the exciting early days of my veterinary career when there were fewer demands on my time and I was able to give all my energy to helping horses. With eighteen years' experience of busy equine practice behind me, it was wonderful to be reminded that it is the "intent" to heal and the ability to communicate with the horse that so often makes a difference. I found this book spiritually uplifting and recommend it to anyone who wishes to know the horse on a deeper level.'

Sue Devereux BA MRCVS BVSc (Hons)
IVAS Cert Veterinary Acupuncture;
Equine Veterinary Surgeon; author of *The Veterinary Care of the Horse*

'As an American physical therapist with a sub-speciality in animal rehabilitation, I am always interested in meeting people who share enthusiasm and love toward the same field. During one of my teaching tours in April 2000, I was fortunate to spend educational, clinical and personal time with Margrit. As a complementary practitioner for animal health, she explodes with compassion, admiration and respect for each animal she comes into contact with. Margrit's work is a natural facilitation towards personal change and healing on a mental, emotional and physical level. While Margrit emphasises healing to the mind of the animal and its energy field, she also displays her passion for healing the animal–human relationship. Her heart's desire is to encourage people to become "a healing person and not a hurting person for their animals". I am confident you will enjoy Margrit's collected studies of her healing work as you journey into the mind of this compassionate healer.'

Gail Wetzler BS, PT
Physical Therapist with clinic in California; Veterinarian Assistant; Equine Sports Massage Therapist; Developer and CEO of Integrative Therapies in Animal Health; Director of Visceral Manipulation Department, Upledger Institute, USA

'Whenever possible, Margrit generously gives her time and talent to our horses and ponies at the Wilton Group, Riding for the Disabled (RDA). Margrit's gift of healing is awesome. Her attunement with her patient is on every level – spiritual, mental, emotional and physical. As soon as she puts her hands on horses, she tunes in. With her communication abilities, she just "knows" what the horse is feeling and thinking – and the area where the problems are. She then gives the healing to try to resolve it, or points us in the right direction with other specialists. It is a great privilege to have Margrit treat our horses and ponies, and to see the calmness in their eyes is to know just how much they enjoy and appreciate it too. I highly recommend this book to every horse owner – it is unique in its insights and information on why we all need to give healing regularly to our horses.'

Pat Burgess
RDA and jumping instructor

'Healer may be a term often associated with someone claiming to be a miracle worker and usually scoffed at not only by scientists, but also by most down-to-earth people. However, the more I work with my hands the more I believe that there really is some energy force that can greatly enhance the normal healing process both physically and emotionally.

'I have met Margrit Coates several times and had the privilege of observing her at work on horses. In my view, she is a powerful facilitator of the release of blocked energy. What is more, she has a very practical approach, works in conjunction with vets, and actively encourages owners to follow the conventional veterinary route. She keeps her mind open to other therapies as well. I would not hesitate to recommend her to anyone with a horse who needs a boost or is suffering from past trauma.'

Catherine Davison ITEC ESMA
Equine Sports Massage Association

'Margrit has become a valuable friend and colleague. We both regularly work together on the same cases and as a result I have been given the opportunity to experience and observe the effects of her healing treatments on horses.

'Some of the cases we have seen responded in ways I never could have imagined. When Margrit has seen them I find my treatments are more effective and longer lasting. Margrit's insight into the horse allows more information to be available and presents me with a greater variety of skills to employ.

'Above all, Margrit has opened up paths for myself and helped to develop my own potential to treat and maintain equilibrium and a healthy status in our animals. This book will make you laugh and cry, but will show you a way to find empathy in your own animal and, if you are a professional, with all your clients. It is a must for all horse carers world wide.'

Amanda Sutton MCSP, SRP, Grad. Dip. Phys.
Chartered Animal Physiotherapist; British Three Day Event team physiotherapist Atlanta Olympic Games 1996

1
The path to the horse within

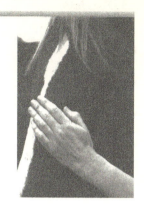

'Out of the depths I have cried to Thee, O Lord
Lord, hear my voice
Let Thine ears be attentive
To the voice of my supplication'
                        Psalm 130 De Profundis

IN THE BEGINNING I thought that everyone could hear it – the horse's voice. Some of the places I went to, where there were lots of horses, the noise could be deafening, a mixture of some shouting, some whispering and some pleading with a haunting echo. They all had different things to say, sometimes a lot of words, sometimes a few, but always quite clearly and emphatically. There was one very handsome bay cob who wasn't being ridden and was offered to me on loan. Harry stood watching me thoughtfully as I approached him in the field. I stood in front of him and, as usual, made a contact on his neck and said hello. At first Harry didn't say anything, just watched me as his owner chatted about things in general. Then suddenly there was a strong eye contact between the horse and myself, which seemed to suspend us in time. He then quite clearly communicated to me that he was a laid back sort of chap but he didn't suffer fools gladly. I mentioned this to the owner and with a look of amazement he asked how I knew this about the horse. The answer was, because he could communicate and I could hear him.

    Not all healers have the gift of extra-sensory contact but this ability and healing attunement was something I first became aware of when I was three years old. I vividly remember sensing things that others couldn't, seeing colours around living creatures and feeling heat and tingling in my hands when I touched sick animals and people. As time went on and I grew up I usually kept these things to myself, for I soon realised that I had unusual gifts and didn't want to be ridiculed. The world was not yet at a stage where energy medicine and healing was acceptable to a wide audience.

Both my parents had hands-on healing abilities and there is also a long history of ancestors on my mother's side who practised medicine and had interests in herbs and homeopathy. My mother came from north-eastern Europe, the daughter of a farmer who bred Trakhener horses, and the deep sense of tradition and culture that I was brought up with and the link to generations of my family who had a close rapport with nature no doubt added to my sensitivity. My grandparents' 1000-acre farm was in East Prussia, just two miles from the Lithuanian border, and as the Russian army invaded towards the end of the Second World War they buried their possessions in the garden, set the livestock free and fled across Europe to northern Germany.

My mother married a Yorkshireman from Hull, where I was born, and as a child I was told many stories of the beloved animals including horses, and worse still of relatives I would never see who were left behind, missing or trapped behind the Iron Curtain. All this had a profound effect on me and nurtured an inborn sensitivity, and a desire developed to help people and animals, somewhere, somehow, one day. Our family were poor when I was a child and riding horses was something that I dreamt of but had to wait for until I was earning a living to achieve. I collected endless books and pictures on horses and when I saw them I would always be compelled to softly touch them, and people would usually notice a calmness come over them – the seed of my healing was in place.

Coming into contact with horses

I started riding in earnest in my twenties, when I was able to realise my dream to learn properly, and I went to dressage trainer and rider Andrew Murphy, who specialises in classical riding. His chestnut gelding schoolmaster Lysander gave me some wonderful lessons and taught me what dancing with a horse means. By this method I learnt physical attunement when riding the horse, which in turn strengthened my mental attunement.

As time went on and I experienced contact with a wide variety of places and equines I genuinely thought that what I could see and feel from the horse was normal. In my innocence I would say things like, 'We shouldn't use that one today, he's got an ache in the hip,' or 'That one is sad and needs some emotional help.' People didn't seem to know what I was talking about and told me to get on and ride them and kick on or give them a smack if they were a problem. I was made to feel awkward and difficult but the worst thing of all was riding a horse who was asking for help and no one was listening. Many people spent a lot of time training to meet the horse's physical needs but neglected the horse within. The horse had to earn its keep or do a job or perform and it was treated like a machine. I spent a lot of my time wandering around the stables laying my hands on these horses to help them have a better sense of wellbeing and find some peace. In those days, the holistic approach for horses was far less acceptable than today so I would often keep what I was doing to myself.

I vividly remember Charlie Brown, a pretty eight-year-old bay gelding who belonged to a riding school that I started going to. The yard owner didn't like him very much, complaining that she found him difficult and moody, and that he bucked. I had stood with him many times in his stable offering him healing because I knew he had a bad left shoulder pain and frequent headaches. I had mentioned it to the owner who scoffed and told me she was the expert, not me. One day the cob I usually rode was out on a hack and Charlie Brown was tacked up ready for my lesson. His eyes bore into mine as I approached and he begged me to help him because he hurt so much. I told the instructor that I wouldn't ride him because he was not well at which she lost her temper and told me to get on. To my everlasting shame she intimidated me to the point where I decided I was perhaps wrong and put my toe in the stirrup to mount the horse. Charlie Brown turned his head suddenly and nipped my foot, a reaction to his pain and the only way he could tell the world at large that he needed help. The instructor lashed him across the mouth with her whip. 'I'm not having a vicious horse in my yard,' she said. Charlie Brown stood rock still with a look of shock and pain on his gentle face. I dismounted, told her what I thought of her and left the place for good, always to wonder what happened to troubled Charlie Brown.

Someday, I told myself, things would change and people would take a step forward in their relationship with the horse and cross a boundary into a more spiritual dimension that would also enrich their own lives. When this happened I knew the partnership of human and horse would be improved for the benefit of both. At least these days I am in a position to officially help horses like Charlie Brown and people are becoming increasingly aware that horses are more than just flesh and bone and are the most sensitive of animals, with a strong emotional side. Times have changed, especially in the last couple of years, and a search for enlightenment is increasing. People are starting to want to return to a depth of inner knowledge and awareness that our ancestors had and that lies dormant in each one of us. It is a dimension that modern man has sacrificed along the way to a material and egotistical evolution. However, it is truly never too late for our spiritual self to emerge from deep within us, and this is where the healing begins. We only have to listen.

A time of questioning

Several years ago I sat in the boardroom of a very luxurious building and yet again felt the niggling pangs of discontentment. I had a lot of material things that went with the high-powered job I was doing but I was finding it more and more difficult to reconcile my career with the development I had done as a healer many years before. In my darkest hour in the late seventies, as I suffered from the backlash of a divorce, I decided to develop my spiritual side and spent three years as a probationary healer with an organisation in Chatham, Kent. The catalyst was an incredible experience I'd had one day, which gave me evidence of the existence of a great power – God. At the time it was a lifeline, something to focus on, but it became the foundation of my future and sent me on a journey of development of deep inner consciousness, which lasted nearly ten years.

I knew that one day I would put the healing I developed during this period to good use but didn't know in what way. I felt I wanted to work with animals but healing in that field, particularly for horses, was a largely uncharted area. During my development as a healer I realised that I had an exceptionally strong clairvoyant gift and it was this ability that I would later put to good use as an equine communicator.

I lived in Kent for 18 years, before moving to Wiltshire with my work, and found it a very good place to be at that time in terms of spiritual enlightenment. I came across many people there who were interested in healing and I treated both animals and people, giving healing on a voluntary basis during the evenings and weekends as I was very busy with my job. Those years were invaluable, as to be really effective the healer needs to practise over a period of time, building up sufficiently strong self-energy and stamina to be able to really work deeply in the energy fields of others.

A time of business

At the same time as I was developing as a healer I was working hard, and with a diploma in graphic design, I climbed the ladder through the world of advertising and marketing, eventually becoming PR department head for a large company. There were aspects of this job that I absolutely loved. I considered myself extremely lucky that I was paid to spend a lot of time involved with the equestrian field and it was there that pieces of the jigsaw began to come together. My boss, who was the chairman of the company, was Philip Billington, now chairman of the British Equestrian Federation. Philip used to joke when asked what he did for a living that his hobby was his job and his work was the horses and as time went on I considered myself very lucky to have a job which incorporated my own hobby of horses. Philip was at the time heavily involved with the British Show Jumping Association and International League for the Protection of Horses (becoming chairman of both eventually) and several other equestrian ventures and charities. So it was for me a dream job as I helped to organise many equestrian events.

When I joined, it was just three UK companies but rapidly expanded to 14 world-wide. One of the original companies manufactured protective industrial clothing and one day during a visit to the factory Philip had an idea. He'd spotted a gap in the market for fashionable weatherproof equestrian clothing and together with advice from several competitors had some prototypes made up. A sample range was put together and tested by various riders until the point was reached a year later, in 1992, where Philip took the decision to form a separate company, and I was very excited to be involved with the launch of the new venture. At the end of one long meeting Philip said to me, 'By the way, it'll need a name, something catchy. Put your mind to it.'

For days I sat at my desk scribbling on bits of paper and flicking through clothing magazines for ideas and inspiration. I wanted something global, descriptive, catchy and, of course, inoffensive in any language. The name came to me suddenly late one sunny afternoon. I wrote it down: 'Toggi'. The company was to be a big and important part of my life for the next five years, during which time I played a central role on behalf of Chemring in the development of Toggi, which went on to become a major clothing brand. Throughout the following years the company was involved in the sponsorship of many riders and top events, including the

Horse of the Year Show at Wembley, Olympia, the Toggi Show Jumping Championships at Stoneleigh and Blenheim Horse Trials.

It was in the autumn of 1992 that Philip invited me to join him for an evening meeting at a large equestrian centre. He had an idea to sponsor a young but recently successful rider, who he felt would go right to the top and be a great ambassador for Toggi. 'This young man is going to be probably the best rider in the world,' he said as we waited in a cold ante-room. He told me his name, but to my embarrassment I'd never heard of him. A shy young man entered the room and shook my boss's hand. He offered him a glass of champagne and turning to me he said, 'I'd like you to meet Blyth Tait.' A New Zealander based in the UK, Blyth was still celebrating winning the Three-Day Event World Championship with his legendary horse Messiah and had approached Philip for sponsorship. That night a deal was struck for Toggi to sponsor Blyth and his horses. Some of the happiest times for me over the next few years were watching him demonstrate his natural and inspiring horsemanship as he climbed the ladder to become the multiple champion that he is today.

Blyth Tait's Messiah

One of the many highlights for me of sponsoring Blyth was having a lesson on the wonderful Messiah. The place where he was stabled at the time had a huge indoor school and when I arrived, Blyth was riding Messiah in there. I sat and watched for more than thirty minutes and, as always, Blyth made it look so easy and effortless, the horse's movements just flowing. He eventually turned to me and said, 'Right. Your turn now,' and pulled the horse up. I mounted and from that day to this have never experienced a sensation like sitting on that horse. It was like the feeling you must get when you drive a Formula One racing car after a family saloon. Messiah hummed with incredible energy and fitness. The lesson started well enough, but the athletic horse was out of my league and he knew it. Within a few minutes we had lost the trot and it became faster and faster until he was carting me around the arena – still at a trot. 'Slow the trot down with your body – don't touch his mouth, he'll get worse,' Blyth shouted to me as I hurtled past at breakneck speed. That was no easy thing to do and I was very relieved when Blyth said, 'I think we'll leave the canter for today.' I just knew that we would have beaten the indoor speed record.

Toggi also sponsored other riders, including event rider Mary King and show jumper Tim Stockdale, and I was relieved that all the Toggi sponsored riders had happy yards. The company also had a presence at numerous trade stands so I was very busy organising things and travelling around shows at all levels of competition. I enjoyed some wonderful days and evenings watching equestrian events and also enjoying the trappings that company sponsorship brings – lavish entertaining in hospitality suites meeting many famous personalities. However, it used to prick my conscience that many of the horses I saw had problems and weren't happy. I knew something could be done about it and that I could help.

A deepening awareness

I came into contact with horses and ponies from a wide variety of disciplines who had lots to say and many who needed hands-on healing. It struck me how much more many people would enjoy their horses and how much better they would do if they were helped with healing treatments. Healing allows a horse the opportunity to experience peace, balance and harmony in an unnatural environment and a stressed world, and to let go of negative energy, offering a chance of improved wellbeing. When I had some free time I would go round the stable areas or horseboxes and talk to the horses, laying my hands on them and offering some healing. I could see that many were greatly relieved to feel the peaceful energy flow and I felt better able to go back and enjoy a glass of champagne knowing I had helped a horse or two feel better.

From the late seventies, when I first developed as a healer, up to that moment, I practised healing on a low-key basis, giving treatments to family and friends and similarly to their animals, including horses. I had deliberately not discussed this healing work with any of my business colleagues or contacts. It would have been confusing for them and unprofessional. Also I didn't want to be accused of using the contacts I had to do something radically different, I wanted to do it on my own merits and because what I did worked for horses. Happier horses would mean happier people and the results would speak for themselves. It just wasn't compatible with my official career at that time and so I kept my own counsel, waiting for the right time to change my life. As time went on I felt that I should somehow be involved with the welfare of horses but my pathway was still hidden in the future. The rumblings of change came in 1995 when my husband Peter went into hospital to have a lump removed from behind his ear, just a cyst we were told. The operation lasted nearly five hours as a huge tumour was found in the parotid (salivary) gland and ten days later the biopsy confirmed our worst fears as cancer was diagnosed.

At that time, none of the cancer organisations had any useful information on alternative therapies and I did my own research. Within a couple of weeks I had become an expert on complementary therapies and what could help during the traumatic period of post-operative recuperation. I found qualified therapists from a wide range of disciplines (herbalism, homeopathy, cranial osteopathy, reflexology and aromatherapy) and I started my own healing treatments on my husband with a vengeance. The hospital where my husband was being treated was not merely sceptical but very much against him using complementary treatment alongside his orthodox treatment. We adopted the approach that his body belonged to him, not the hospital, and carried on.

Each evening I would give Peter lengthy healing treatments and he would have some marvellous responses – his wounds healed much more quickly than anyone expected. I knew that he would be OK and this was confirmed when a few months later he was given the all clear. His consultant admitted when he discharged him that he was amazed at how well he had done considering the severity of the operation and the radiotherapy to his face area. The other therapies that I had come into contact with fascinated me and I wanted to learn more about anatomy and physiology of both humans and animals. Overnight I knew that I wanted to be a practitioner of complementary medicine but how do you give up everything when you are in your late forties and the household's major breadwinner? Things were changing on the work front, however – separate management had been brought in to run Toggi and as a result I was becoming less involved as time went on. The rest of the company's products were not nearly as interesting for me and for the next two years I felt a definite pull away from what I was doing, a restlessness growing inside me as I spent more and more time thinking about my healing roots.

Making the move

Often when we are ready for change and feel that our lives should follow a different direction, we get little signposts along the way. At around this

THE PATH TO THE
HORSE WITHIN

time such a pointer was flagged up in front of me. It was late summer in 1996 that Blyth threw a huge party at his home to celebrate winning two medals at the Atlanta Olympic Games – individual gold and team bronze. Tables and chairs had been put on the lawn and a trestle table was brimming with the most delicious food. Crates of champagne lined the entrance hall to the house and Blyth's two medals had pride of place on a small table next to the gate of a paddock in which his winning horses Ready Teady and Chesterfield were grazing. They had just a few days before returned from the US and were in very frisky form, and how typical of Blyth that he should turn the now very valuable horses out to relax and play and 'be horses'.

Some of my colleagues from Toggi were with me and we shared a table enjoying the warm summer evening and wonderful scenery. Also seated at the table was a very distinguished businessman called Ralf, who I had not previously met. We all talked about things in general and then I got talking to Ralf about life on a more in-depth level. He suddenly turned to me and said, 'You are a healer, aren't you?' At this my workmates looked up in anticipation of my answer. I felt embarrassed and didn't answer. Ralf stood up to leave. 'You are a healer and you should go back to your roots, there is much work for you to do.' He waved his hand in the direction of the horses as he walked away. I felt the hairs stand up on the back of my neck and not wanting to discuss it with the others at the table quickly changed the subject. This man's comments had a big effect on me and I couldn't get his words out of my head. I became more and more restless, knowing that a sign had been flagged up, but not knowing in which direction I should go.

It was one morning in early April 1997 that I reached my crossroads and my desire for change was answered. It was one of those occasions that at the time we wish we hadn't asked for because when it comes it is so dramatic.

Philip called me into his office and I noticed that he looked upset and shaky. The personnel manager was with him and he explained that several overseas investments had depleted the group's cash flow and drastic restructuring had been ordered by the board. The head office of which I was part was to lose most of its staff as companies were to be sold off. Redundancy negotiations began. I walked out of his office and felt that a huge weight had lifted from me and that the next and most important and exciting phase of my life could begin.

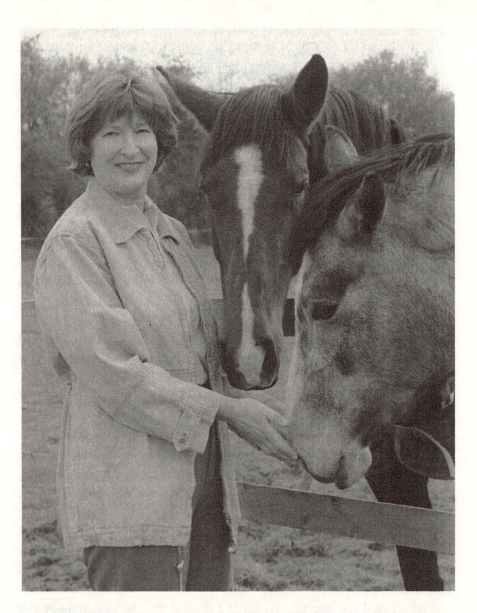

Margrit Coates with Casini and Rouella.

At this time I also saw a course advertised for a qualification in anatomy and physiology, which was a prerequisite for other qualifications in complementary therapies, and I enrolled. Thus started a period of intensive study and exams until I was able to set up my own practice offering a range of treatments as well as healing. There were many times when the money nearly ran out but once I started I knew this was what I had really wanted to do all my life. One of the major benefits of my studying was that

THE PATH TO THE
HORSE WITHIN

it gave me scientific answers to the responses and reactions that I got when giving healing treatments and helped me to understand energy medicine. You can say that I put the cart before the horse in that I had been doing the work before I had the technical knowledge to explain it.

Eventually I was thrilled to be able to extend my equestrian background by attending specialist workshops including equine cranio-sacral therapy with Gail Wetzler, who came over to the UK from California to run her unique course. After I had become a full-time animal healer I phoned Ralf and asked him about the message that he had given to me. He remembered the conversation very well but didn't know why he had said what he did, the words had just seemed to come to him. He was very pleased that his words had had such a very profound effect on me and told me that my phone call had made his day.

It was at the time of my new beginning that my healing work for horses took off in a big way. A couple of years before, I had met dressage judge and instructor Gillian Makey Harfield at Penton Horse Trials when I was writing notes for her as she judged a competition, and one day just after my redundancy she phoned me. 'Can you come over to the yard?' she asked. 'I'm having lots of problems with all my boys so thought that some of your healing sessions could help.' Gill runs a livery yard in Dorset and I took myself over there to treat her five horses. A couple of days after my visit she contacted me to say she was thrilled with the improvements to all of them and was passing my name on to other riders with problems. At the same time I was asked by another contact to visit the horse of a friend of hers near where I live to give it healing. This was also very successful and she began to recommend me to other riders and owners. From then onwards requests for me to treat horses with healing snowballed to the point where in a short period of time I was treating more horses than humans. My path then took another very important turn.

Top to Toe

I was frequently seeing horses who were communicating physical problems. The healing could help but in some of the cases an extra dimension was needed for the conditions that some of the horses had. I was aware of all the complementary therapies available for people and used a physiotherapist and osteopath for my own back problems. Where could I find someone highly qualified and competent that I could recommend to horses' owners? Being properly qualified and working with vet permission were paramount as horses are vulnerable to unregulated people who profess to have skills that they do not. At least humans can speak up for themselves if a practitioner hurts them or makes them feel worse and can refuse to see them again. But the horse has no such control over his destiny and can only suffer in silence. Using someone unqualified means at the very least that an owner/rider could be wasting their money and at worst having their horse's problems made very much worse.

I got in touch with Gill Makey Harfield as I knew that having competed at a top level she would know who was bona fide and who was not. She mentioned a person who she used to treat her own horses and who, in fact, I had heard of and seen at work from a distance at some of the horse trial events I had been to with Toggi – Amanda Sutton. Amanda was the British Three Day Event team equine physiotherapist at the 1996 Olympic Games in Atlanta and I knew she was very highly regarded. So I contacted her office, got some of her leaflets and starting passing her details on to owners when I thought it appropriate, notably for musculo-skeletal problems.

One day the phone rang and it was Amanda. She said she was amazed by things that owners were telling her about improvements to their horses after healing from me and she wanted to meet up with me. She was also finding that when we treated animals together (although at different times) she often got quicker results. The week she rang I was due to visit a large equine rehabilitation centre near Oxford and she asked if she could watch me treat the horses there. We met in a little village tea shop and over lunch talked about our work and plans for the future. It was wonderful to find that we had so much in common with a mutual vision to improve the welfare of the horse. As we talked, ideas began to form and I knew that our meeting was the beginning of something very profound and special. After lunch we went to the rehabilitation stables and I treated several horses (see Chapter 5: Case histories and page 13). At the end of the day, Amanda turned to me and said, 'If you'd like to work together we could do some courses at my yard. Perhaps you'd like to think about it?' I was very excited at the opportunity to expand and form a team for the good of the horse and over the next few weeks an idea was born.

Loving and free

It was during one of my visits to an equine rehabilitation centre that something very profound happened. The last horse of the day who was brought out for me to treat was a piebald called Tony. He wasn't the world's prettiest horse but from his eye shone real depth of character and intelligence. Tony was strong and unruly and he dragged his groom along the corridor as she led him towards me. The horse stopped next to me and as we looked at each other I could see intense suffering in his aura. I could see pictures showing lots of ropes around him, also a longing for food and water, and as I tuned in to the horse's past his feelings became mine – I was starving and lonely and no one came to help me.

By this time Tony was settling down and I decided to start giving him some healing. The horse resisted for a while, ready to move off if he didn't like what was happening. Then suddenly peace came over him and those staring eyes flickered and closed. His head nodded and he sighed, swinging his back and resting first one leg then another. The atmosphere around us became heavy and everything seemed far away. In the distance I could hear the barking of the rescue dogs from their compound but then that faded too. I stepped forward and raising my hand gently placed it on to the front of Tony's head. The horse looked at me softly – his eye was only a couple of inches from mine and now the look from him was one not of fear but of love. As our eyes made contact I felt as though as I were looking into the eyes of God, our souls meeting in a suspension of time and place. It also seemed that I knew everything about the universe, in that moment, in that look. Then I heard the song. It slipped into my mind and I was singing it before I realised. 'Loving and free,' the words went. The tune was vaguely familiar but it was the words that seemed important. 'I will untangle myself so that I can see, I will untangle myself so that I can be loving and free.'

Tony's eye continued to mesmerise my own and we remained locked in our sacred communication. After a while I realised that a long time had passed and reluctantly I prepared to take my hand away. It was difficult, though, it seemed drawn to the horse as though it were magnetised. Tony sighed and then started to lick and chew in acceptance. The moment had passed but still I could hear the song. The horse started to get restless and, wanting some air myself, I followed the groom out as he was put into a paddock. I asked the groom if she knew the song which had come to me, but she didn't.

Back in the staff room over a coffee we discussed Tony's history. He had been at the centre for about eight months and was the subject of an RSPCA prosecution case, having been brought in with a pony. Both had been neglected and Tony was terrified of dark places so possibly he had been shut in somewhere. All the way home, quite a long drive, the song bugged me – I couldn't identify it yet it seemed the words would have a special message. The first thing I did when I entered my front door was sing it to my husband. 'What is this song?' I asked. 'It's driving me mad.' 'Oh, I know that,' he said, 'we've got it on a CD.' A few minutes later the song was playing: 'Loving and Free' by Kiki Dee. I explained to my husband what had happened that day and we both wept as we listened to the words.

I phoned after two days to ask about Tony and his groom said a big breakthrough had happened. Tony was immediately more relaxed after I had treated him but one particular thing stood out. The horse had always been difficult to catch and during the eight months that Tony had been at the centre he had led the staff a merry dance when they went to bring him in from the paddocks, taking two to three hours to be caught every time. They noticed that he was much more relaxed about being caught after the healing and suddenly, the day after my visit, came the biggest change. It was time to bring the horses in and Tony stood still as his groom approached him in the field, not turning away as she walked up to him. He walked happily in as though he didn't have a care in the world and from then onwards he was very easy to catch.

From time to time when giving healing to very troubled horses I hear this song in my mind and I know then that some very special and powerful healing is taking place.

Loving and Free

Bound I am bound like the knots in a string
Eager to be where my life can begin

Out of the shadow and into the sun
So many things that I should have done

I will untangle myself so that I can see
I will untangle myself, everything will be – loving and free

Bound I am bound like a rope on a swing
Up in the air and then down again

Sure for the first time, so clear in my mind
Wise to the feeling I gently unwind

I will untangle myself so that I can see
I will untangle myself, everything will be – loving and free

Bound I am bound to remember your smile
Something so special doesn't fade away

Sadness is sweet when you're gone for a while
When I see you there'll be a lot to say

I will untangle myself so that I can see
I will untangle myself, everything will be – loving and free

Written and performed by Kiki Dee

Amanda and I put together a programme in which owners would bring their horses for the day to have a health check and rebalance. I had felt for a long time that everything on offer was still geared very much for the benefit of the rider and that the horse was secondary. Even the newly emerging natural methods of training were asking the horse to do something that the human dictated and the voice of the horse and its inner needs were frequently overlooked. Training was often put on top of emotional and or physical problems, which were not resolved. I felt we should offer something where we listened to the horse, what remedies it needed, where it had aches and pains and where the animal could be rebalanced with healing. We needed to find out what was necessary to make the horse happy on a much deeper level. After a great deal of discussion, Amanda and I put together a package that combined the different disciplines of physiotherapy, dentistry, saddle fitting, veterinary homeopathy and healing – all on the same day and in the same place. It was a unique concept and we very quickly filled the five places on offer, for this, our first, Top to Toe Day. We considered that the homeopathy element was very important for our philosophy of helping the horse on a deeper level and for our first Top to Toe Day we had holistic vet Nick Thompson as our official veterinary controller. The event took place on a crisp but sunny spring day and it proved so popular that we now run Top to Toe Days every month at our practice near Winchester.

Holistic Pets and Help for Horses

Very quickly we were approached by people who requested natural treatments for their dog and cats, as well as other animals, and we realised we needed to expand to fulfil this need and have a regular vet on board. Another piece of the jigsaw fell in to place when we met homeopathic vet Cheryl Sears at a lecture. She was an independent vet with a regular popular BBC radio slot who was looking to take her skills to a wider audience, so we all got together to plan our next step. After several meetings we had the plan in place, a unique clinic offering natural treatments for animals, which we named Holistic Pets. The clinic has a treatment room for small animals as well as a large horse treatment room and people can choose from homeopathy, physiotherapy or healing for their animals. In a short period of time, Holistic Pets became very popular and it now receives frequent referrals from a number of vets. We thought that we had realised our vision but it didn't stop there.

It became apparent that many horses had such a lot of problems that they needed specialist residential care. Our practice near Winchester is in a beautiful rural setting with plenty of comfortable stabling, large post and rail paddocks, a round pen, an all-weather menage and, of course, the treatment rooms. So we thought how we could best continue to serve the interest of the horse and the next logical step for us was to set up Help for Horses. Owners can send their horses to our facility for rehabilitation for whatever period of time suits them best. They can choose from a comprehensive programme of specialist care for their horse to cover physical and emotional rehabilitation. As well as healing from me, homeopathy and herbs from Cheryl and physiotherapy from Amanda and her team, there are other experts we associate with who share our philosophy of treating the horse holistically and can treat the horse while it is at the centre. These include practitioners in natural methods of backing and schooling, classical riding, team work for both horse and rider, massage therapy, nutritional advice, veterinary acupuncture, cranio-sacral therapy, osteopathy, dentistry and saddle fitting.

The welfare of the horses during their residential care at Help for Horses is, of course, under the watchful supervision of a vet from the local equine practice, who conveniently also keeps her own horse at the yard and is very keen on holistic horsemanship. A wide variety of horses can benefit from this facility, including the injured, those who have had illness or surgery, those suffering from trauma, the newly acquired with problems and those that develop them, the young horse and the rescued horse. Of course, the horse doesn't even have to be injured or have particular problems to spend time at the centre. We have taken horses as a 'health cure' to give them a good holiday and improve their wellbeing and we are also used by people who are travelling or going through a busy period who want their horses to be holistically cared for.

From my point of view, one of the key elements to the effective working of these disciplines is healing, because if the horse's energy field is in balance then everything else has a better chance of success. Healing can provide a foundation that other therapies can build on and link to. Giving the horse the chance to feel at peace is a very gratifying part of the rehabilitation process.

The opportunities and demands for my healing work with horses are growing incredibly quickly, beyond all my expectations. It seems that people are ready now, at the start of the twenty-first century, to take a step forward in their relationship with that noblest of animals – the horse.

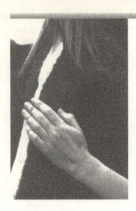

2
What is healing for horses?

'Final and complete healing will come from within, from the soul itself, which by His beneficence radiates harmony throughout the personality when allowed to do so.'
Dr Edward Bach

THE THERAPY OF HEALING by using the hands as a channel for energy into the spirit of a person or animal is the oldest form of medicine and goes back to the beginning of time. Healing is older even than the use of plants and herbs, which are the forerunners of modern medicine, and ancient paintings and drawings show people laying their hands on others. Indian Vedic texts more than 2000 years old describe universal energy and how this is channelled deep into the cells of a human body through energy centres called chakras. In Egyptian temples the priests used their hands to give healing to the sick, and the touch of hands for this reason has continued through the ages in many different cultures. The concept of life force energy is shared by many of the world's long-established and ancient medicines, which use this force for healing. For example, in Japanese medicine it's called ki, in Chinese traditional medicine it's called chi, in Ayurveda it's prana and the Greeks called it pneuma.

Within every living being lies the life force or essence of the body – the spirit. It is a vibrant, oscillating field of energy and healing aims to direct a positive flow to this life force and thereby release negative energy. It has been scientifically shown that as the universe pulsates with energy, so each cell in a body vibrates and is in a constant state of dynamic change. Modern science has done a great deal of research into energy and through this we know that all things on the earth, living or otherwise, are part of a complete system of energy, including cosmic. These forces influence us and our horses every second of every day. Where there is a problem in the body, lesions or blockages occur in the energy field and the centres of energy within that body start to vibrate out of rhythm. It is not just the physical condition but also the emotional state that affect this field.

I have found that healing for the horse can be very successful at stimulating the release of deep memory and emotional blockage within cells and tissues, and even in the life force itself. Where does this negative and chaotic energy go? Into the universe for it to deal with.

When I place my hands on a horse I feel as though I am picking up all the instruments in an orchestra, most of which are out of tune – these are, of course, all the energy imbalances in the body. Every cell in the horse's body has a resonant frequency that gives off certain energy interactive 'notes'. During the course of the treatment I am busily picking up these 'notes' and 'tuning the instruments' until I am playing a symphony. Then I know I have achieved homeostasis, or the best balance possible, for that horse.

Hands-on healing

The healing that this book covers is what I call 'true healing' – laying the hands on to a body to channel healing energy. It is often called spiritual healing. The word spirit means vital animating essence of a person or animal, so the term spiritual healing means universal healing of that vital essence within the body. There are no symbols (as in Reiki for example), rituals or dogma to follow. It is a form of healing that no one can lay claim to having discovered or invented for it is as ancient as our world and belongs to each and every one of us; each man woman and child of the universe who chooses to be a healing person rather than a hurting person. Healing is healing and doesn't need to be reinvented, have a new set of rules or have a distracting title. The potential and power is there to be discovered within us all each day and to be followed as a way of life. 'True healing' is done on a one-to-one basis – involving an exchange of energy between the healer, the one receiving it (e.g. the horse) and the creator (spiritual source) – and it is gentle and non-invasive. There is no hierarchy to follow; it is your own personal relationship with the healing power. The supposed trouble spot may not be where the source of the problem lies and for this reason healers usually treat on a general level, allowing the body to take the healing energy wherever it is needed. The actual source of the problem may lie deep in the horse and could have been triggered off a long time ago, often many years before the current condition appeared.

'We all have a choice – to be a healing person or a hurting person.'
Margrit Coates

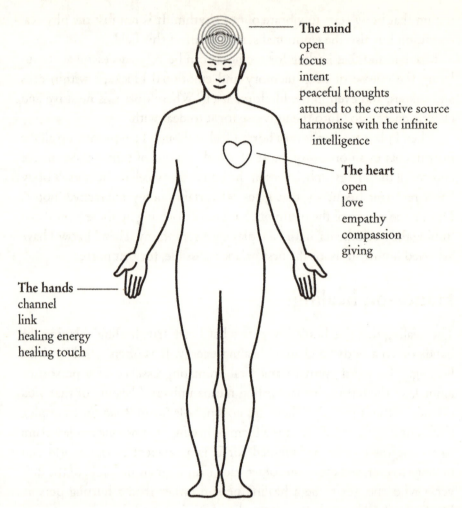

The mind
open
focus
intent
peaceful thoughts
attuned to the creative source
harmonise with the infinite intelligence

The heart
open
love
empathy
compassion
giving

The hands
channel
link
healing energy
healing touch

The healer
Healers use physical energy (via the hands), mental energy (with the mind) and emotional energy (through love) to treat the horse holistically. The illustration shows some key words for healing.

By strengthening the horse's body with healing and by achieving homeostasis it is hoped that the horse will respond and begin to repair or stabilise from within. Healing can work emotionally, mentally or physically and during a treatment energy is transferred via the healer to the animal and travels down lines of energy in the horse's body. These lines of energy may correspond to chakras and meridians (see page 21) or they may not. I have found that in reality I can place my hands anywhere on the horse and start a healing effect although often I target specific areas where I touch, based on my experience. When we give healing to a horse we are creators of beneficial and positive energy – it allows us to release destructive energy into the universe for it to deal with.

Chakras, meridians and electromagnetic fields

Chakras are whirlpools of energy found in various parts of the body and relate to physical, emotional and mental health. Chakras are linked one to the other and have a negative and positive polarity. Energy from the chakras can be felt by the hands and sensitive individuals can also see colours emitted from them. I describe each chakra and its benefits more fully in Chapter Seven.

Meridians are pathways in the body along which the vital energy force flows. These meridians emit light and can be seen using infrared photography.

An electromagnetic field surrounds and penetrates the physical body and influences what happens on the physical level. These fields can be photographed and filmed. Study of electromagnetic qualities has shown they are associated with channels and energy points throughout the body. Similarly, an energy field is radiated outwards from the earth and is called the geomagnetic field.

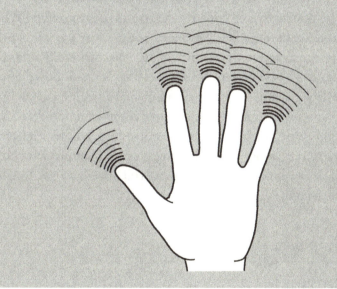

Pulsing magnetic fields are emitted from the hands of healers to scan through the horse to help on whatever level needs healing. Electromagnetic pulses channel universal healing energy to the horse.

The healer uses his or her own electromagnetic field to channel in healing energy but it is something extra that actually creates the healing, a powerful, potent and mysterious force greater than mankind. This rebalancing of the horse's energy field stimulates the animal's own inner resources to

The horse

| physical | mental | emotional |

Hands-on healing aims to help on all levels by restoring balance, or homeostasis.

Imbalance in any of these areas can lead to illness, disease and behavioural problems.

become activated, allowing a return to a situation where everything within the horse works in harmony. Some healers say that they draw the healing energy into their own body before it passes on to the person or animal in need. I personally don't do this, instead having evolved a method that works better for me (see page 109). As I touch the horse to begin healing, my energy field pulsing through my fingertips only at that instant makes a link with the universal energy and joins that to the horse.

Energy can be destructive or constructive, positive or negative. When energy is destructive or negative it changes body tissue for the worse; when energy is constructive or positive it has the power to heal and change body tissue for the better. Within the body's tissue flows something more subtle yet again – emotional and mental energies and energies of the soul. Healing aims to rebalance all these complex, interrelated and interacting energies for the benefit of the horse as a whole. The most important thing to remember is that healing is more than just an adjustment of energy. It is a link to a higher force, which we have yet to truly discover or understand.

My definition of healing

The healer is the channel for the spiritual force of universal healing energy. This source provides the electromagnetic fingerprint, or blueprint, to match what is missing in the horse. This energy is channelled to the horse at the deepest levels by the healer – and can work physically, mentally or emotionally.

WHAT IS HEALING
FOR HORSES?

Our healing focus

The healer's intent and thoughts are most important during a healing treatment. Inside our skulls we have a brain that is responsible for all the functions of the body. The brain produces four energy frequency ranges – alpha, beta, delta and theta – and researchers have demonstrated that during the deep concentration and relaxation achieved by healers, their brains usually have all four wave states operating at once. Renowned British psychologist Maxwell Cade, who invented the machine that records these waves, calls this the 'awakened mind' and the more that people practise healing, the easier and quicker they find it to enter. Usually people don't have all four wave frequencies operating at once. Alpha waves link the conscious and subconscious mind; beta waves are the normal waking state of thinking and problem solving; delta are the waves produced during deep sleep or meditation; and theta are waves of the dreaming or inspirational mind.

During a healing treatment, brain wave patterns of both the healer and the receiver have been shown to synchronise in the alpha state. Also during healing these synchronised brain wave patterns pulse in unison with the earth's magnetic field, known as the Schumann Resonance. So we

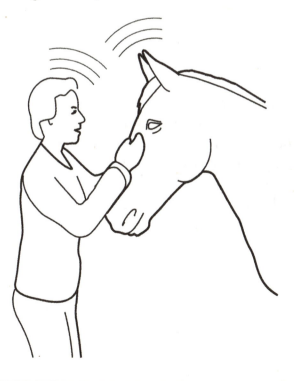

Brain wave patterns of healers pulse in unison with the earth's magnetic field, known as the Schumann Resonance. Research has shown that the wave patterns of healer and receiver synchronise in the alpha state, characteristic of meditation and deep relaxation.

can see how important our mental focus is during the time we give healing to our horse and what extra energy the horse can pick up from us. We should be aware that the horse's brain also emits wave patterns, which will be affected by healing, and that is why healing can produce such calmness as the brain releases endorphins during a treatment. Endorphins produce a sedative-like effect and are also nature's painkillers, helping with relief from discomfort.

Within the brain lies our mind, something that no one has ever seen or measured, and no one can say where it actually lies in the brain. The mind is an active field of energy in which all our thoughts live, each thought with an energy of its own. The mind's energy exists outside of the physical body, as does the energy of the horse's mind. The experiments of Dr Cade give us some insight into how powerful and complex our mind energies are and how little we actually still understand or know. When we focus our thoughts to give healing we contact the horse's mental field and likewise it contacts ours. By doing so it can receive great comfort and peace from knowing that we wish to help it.

When the body dies, the energy of the mind continues to exist, including the energies from the minds of our horses. When they have passed away in terrible conditions their fear and anguish creates a darkness in the universe; where they have known love and caring then their happiness lives on as light. So we can see how powerful and potent simply 'thinking healing' becomes and why intent and focus is so important. This creates a means of attaching our electromagnetic field to that of the horse and channelling the healing that is needed through our hands.

When we give healing it is a living and unselfish prayer raising the energy of the world. The giver is enriched and it is generous and beneficial to give healing to our horses even when they appear well rather than wait until problems appear. I often think of a relevant piece from *The Prophet* by Kahlil Gibran:

'You pray in your distress and in your need. Would that you might pray also in the fullness of your joy and in your days of abundance.'

By giving healing we receive healing for we open ourselves up to experience and knowledge on a raised level of consciousness, which ultimately helps us with our everyday lives and our relationship with horses.

WHAT IS HEALING FOR HORSES?

The benefits of healing for horses

- ❖ Healing may be safely used for all conditions and has no adverse side effects.
- ❖ Healing reaches throughout the physical body as well as the mental and emotional state.
- ❖ Healing is a natural therapy and works with the individual horse's body.
- ❖ Healing may be able to succeed when all else has failed.
- ❖ Healing can be used preventatively.
- ❖ Healing can produce a feeling of peacefulness and inner calm.
- ❖ Healing can help other treatments work on a deeper level.
- ❖ Healing is sometimes successful in one treatment, more often a few treatments are needed, the number depending on the condition.

Research and scientific evidence for the success of healing

Energy medicine has become the buzz word of the twenty-first century as though it's something new. But it isn't, it's part of the ancient wisdom. What is new is that we are recognising after a long time in the spiritual wilderness that healing works for horses and other animals as well as for humans, and we now have the scientific means to measure this energy in all its complexities. But it has always been there, in and around us and our horses, and it forms the basis of healing. It doesn't come in a bottle or have to be ordered, we can just step out into the yard at any time and begin to heal and help our horse or pony. Health and vitality for the horse operates from a deep spiritual level, which healing touches at that core.

Until fairly recently, scientists have been quite sceptical about the claims made for hands-on healing but more and more research has produced conclusive proof that healing works on several levels and that it works by using energies. Scientific research has shown that energy fields of oscillating magnetic resonance are emitted from the hands of healers similar to

'A quantum, defined as the basic unit of matter or energy, is from 10,000,000 to 100,000,000 times smaller than the smallest atom. At this level where matter and energy are interchangeable true healing begins.'
Deepak Chopra

that used by pulsed electromagnetic therapy machines used by the medical profession to treat soft tissue or bone injuries. This shows how healing can help to stimulate repair for a horse's injuries alongside conventional veterinary methods of treatment. Further, the electromagnetic fields from healers' hands help stimulate the release of deep memory and emotional blockages within the tissues.

There are many diverse pieces of research into healing and its effects and in 1999 the *Journal of the Royal Society of Medicine* published a paper which found healing to be highly effective. The study covered people with chronic health problems and 81 per cent reported improvements after they were given healing treatments, with those people still feeling better three months later. Early in 2000, researchers from the University of Maryland published their findings from 23 studies into healing and its effects. The evidence demonstrated that healing can reduce pain and speed recovery from illness.

In another study, which took place in 1982, patients with high blood pressure were split into groups, one of which received healing. This group showed a significant improvement in blood pressure compared with the non-healed groups. Healing can speed up the repair of soft tissue and bone and in 1990 a double blind study on wounds was conducted, which showed a marked improvement and repair rate in patients who were given healing. Experiments have been conducted with animals and wound healing – in one such test mice had pieces of skin removed under strict laboratory conditions, and a group who were exposed to healers recovered much more quickly than those who were not. As an animal healer I personally find it distressing and ironic that we have deliberately damaged animals, no matter how small, to prove that healing energies exist. But at least there is now scientific evidence to prove what our ancestors intuitively knew thousands of years ago, and the healing wheel has come full circle.

Several other serious pieces of research over the past fifty years have conclusively shown that the growth of plants can be influenced by healers either by concentrating on them or by laying their hands over them. The pioneer was Dr Bernard Grad from McGill University in Canada. Dr Grad asked a healer to hold in his hands two identical jars containing water. Some barley seeds were divided into two piles and one was watered with the 'healed' water, the other with untreated water. The seeds were left to grow and seven weeks later the seeds given the 'healed' water were much bigger and greener than the other batch as they contained higher levels of chlorophyll.

This experiment was repeated many times and each time the same thing happened. In another experiment, a person who was suffering from severe depression held and concentrated on a jar of water. The seeds which had this water applied didn't grow at all. And this gives us an inkling of how a horse is going to be affected by our state of mind and how our thoughts are going to be so very important to it. It also shows why we should not attempt to give healing to our horses when we are feeling low or depressed.

Other researchers proved that healing can influence haemoglobin, which is biochemically almost identical to chlorophyll. In 1971, Dolores Krieger (an American nurse) and Oscar Estabany (a healer) helped to carry out experiments on patients suffering from a wide variety of illnesses. One group received healing and one did not. In the treated group, haemoglobin levels rose significantly and other long-term benefits were also reported. Krieger went on to teach healing to medical professionals as Therapeutic Touch, now used in hospitals around the world. As a result of extensive medical evidence over the years the National Health Service in the UK lists healing as an official therapy which doctors are permitted to refer patients for. Similarly, the Royal College of Veterinary Surgeons also raises no objection to hands-on healing as a therapy for animals alongside veterinary care. In the US each state has its own veterinary practice act governing the use of complementary therapies, and will give local advice.

The sceptics of healing point to isolated and lonely people and say that healing works because it makes them feel cared for, that someone is giving their problem attention. They say that is why healing is effective, arguing that positive thinking by the patient makes them believe that the healing is effective, i.e. that they convince themselves that they feel better. Well that argument flies right out of the window when talking about giving healing to horses. The horse doesn't see a therapist or healer standing in front of it, it doesn't understand the concept of healing or of energies, that it can be helped this way. It responds to the healing for what it is and what it feels it to be – and the results are there during and after the healing session. In short, there is no placebo effect when healing horses. Results from healing experiments with animals prove that something more than the power of suggestion is happening because animals are not open to the concept of ideas. I have many sceptics come to watch me work and they usually go away with plenty to think about. Sometimes they ponder over whether they imagined what they felt, but the horse's response is very real, and therefore the experience opens up a new perspective for them.

The energy fields in and around us and our horse

The horse's energy field, like our own, consists of a complex interacting and interrelated network. It is a combination of pulsing fields including magnetic, electrical, thermal (heat), light, gravity, kinetic and sound fields. These fields have no boundaries and it is within, and with, all of these fields that a healer works to clear and release blockages in the horse, and to rebalance the flow of energies. Healers may work within a combination of these fields or in all of them simultaneously, depending on the horse's problem at the time.

Scientists have concluded that although the strength of these fields becomes weaker with distance, there isn't a point at which the field actually stops. All of these energy fields are measurable, as is the energy from individual organs, tissues and cells. Depending on which level of energy I am working in when giving healing, different things can be felt. For example, if I'm working in the electrical field, tingling may be felt, heat if I'm working in the thermal field, and twitches in muscles from the kinetic field. Also during healing I have found that the areas over certain meridians can feel more resistant as the light wavelength is stimulated.

The energy frequency coming from a healer's hands pulses and changes constantly as the horse's body responds, and is called the biomagnetic field. During healing, this field has been measured to be at least 1000 times greater than normal. It is the emission of these fields from my hands that my clients pick up as tingling or pulsing when they touch the horse as I am giving it healing. During healing a lot of work is involved from our own energy field, as it is needed to transmit all the frequencies needed by the horse and it will constantly vary the level and intensity of its vibration to match that of the horse and its requirements. The healing energy comes from a source outside the healer, but the healer needs to tune in to his or her own energy field to allow this to happen and that is something that

The spirit of the horse

Within the horse's body, as within our own body, flows a complicated field of energy. Within that field of energy is also something that cannot be measured – the essence, spirit or soul. Some people refer to this life force as chi, the vital force or vital energy, and the source of it is everywhere, both in us and around us, and it is the driving force of the horse. It may sound strange to think of the horse as having a soul, but the soul is that spark of the life force that links the individual to the universal energy. Without that link, quite simply that individual horse wouldn't exist and I know from my extensive healing experience with horses that they do have a spiritual side to them. This spiritual side is inexorably linked to the spiritual nature of humans.

Mankind has often confused the meaning of the word soul and the concept seems to have been often hijacked for exclusive human use but I believe the soul is a combination of mind energy and life-force energy, which exists in all living things. To deny the horse has a soul – a spark of eternal life force – is to block the evolution of our own soul and which surely remains impoverished by the denial. This life-force energy also has a 'memory' of past incidents, accidents and illness and plays a role in the total health picture of the horse. It can be a reason why a horse is out of balance and in need of healing. As an animal communicator, as well as a healer, I am able to pick up these life-force memories together with information from the mind of the horse.

When the horse passes away from this world, that spark leaves and returns to the great divine source in the universe from whence it came. I believe that no one on this earth has the full answer as to what happens next. Several times I have been with an animal giving healing at the time of its physical death and it has been a most bizarre yet spiritually uplifting experience. As I held these animals I have felt a sudden explosion in my hands like an electric shock, and it was once so strong that it nearly knocked me off my feet. This energy flew outwards from the animal's body just as the vet announced the actual passing. I recently felt the life force leave one of my terminally ill cats as he was put to sleep and the sensation was like a tingling, spinning wheel, which rose to a crescendo and then flew outwards. As the

> sensation stopped I knew the cat was clinically dead but the life force was not. His true life, which is the sum total of indestructible energy, had gone to a much higher plane. Energy doesn't stop being energy so somewhere out there that imprint still exists – where and how no one really knows. I have given healing to horses just before their death but not held on to them during it (a very dangerous and difficult thing to do with the horse) so I have not yet felt this explosion or movement of energy in my hands from them. However, there is no reason to think that it would be any different.

some people find easier than others. The concentration needed is tiring and that is why I limit the number of healing treatments that I give in a day.

The aura

Science has been able to demonstrate that surrounding a body is an electrical field – and that includes the body of the horse. This field is called an aura, and sensitive and intuitive people are able to actually see it, either as a series of colours or as a shimmering light. I have seen this energy layer many times as a dense band of white light directly around the body with a less bright light radiating outwards like a pale glow from the moon. It is something I've seen around horses and other animals, sometimes strongly, sometimes weakly, depending on what I was treating the animal for and the strength of its energy field. When I look at a horse it is where I see dark spots or patches in this aura that I know the horse has some sort of problem.

The electrical field (aura) around the body has been photographed in a technique called Kirlian photography, named after a famous Russian scientist. Photography of the human aura has revealed that this, in fact, changes in quality when the psychological and physical condition of the person is altered. The same is going to be true for horses for they vibrate with energy just as we do and also emit an electrical field.

The electrical field of a body extends some way outwards, depending on the extra-sensory development of the individual, and the more healing we do the bigger and stronger it grows. Sometimes when I approach a horse it snorts and blows at me, looking wild-eyed for a moment or two. I know

WHAT IS HEALING FOR HORSES?

it is detecting my strong healing aura and it wonders what that is. Our surrounding electrical field is constantly vibrating, oscillating and moving on many different planes. What is in our mind and our emotions influence the activity within this energy field, so we can see how important our inner thoughts are. This is why we often pick up bad vibes from one person or good vibes from another. The horse is very sensitive to this surrounding electrical field and negative mental or emotional vibes can affect it adversely. Healing thought and intent produces positive electrical energy, which has a beneficial effect on the horse at all levels.

The living matrix

A person giving healing to a horse is not just touching the horse's skin or the energy above the skin, but is getting in touch with a complicated network that extends continuously throughout the horse's body called the living matrix – an interconnected information network, which oscillates and vibrates with life-force energy. The skin is the largest organ of the horse and in my experience frequently shows signs of immediate healing changes during a treatment or shortly after. The skin can become softer or looser, veins may stand out, the coat may become more shiny and small lumps and bumps can flatten. When you touch the horse you are communicating through the living matrix with every cell within its body. What affects one part, at whatever level, affects another and the healing touch aims to bring harmony where there is chaos. The skin is influenced by the autonomic nervous system, further explaining why the deep calming and

Energy fields and healing

- ❖ Living organisms, including the horse, are surrounded by bio-electromagnetic fields.
- ❖ These fields are constantly changing, depending on what is happening to the horse – either emotionally, physically or mentally – giving a picture of what is going on inside its body.
- ❖ When giving healing to a horse it is these fields that I listen to and scan with my hands and mind to pick up where the blockages are.

inner changes which healing triggers are reflected by the relaxation of the skin. The healer links the living matrix of the horse with healing energy from the universal master source.

Distant healing

Healing can be sent over a long distance by thought and by prayer, and experiments conducted by doctors have shown the effects of distant healing. A group of heart patients were sent distant healing (without their knowledge) and they showed dramatic improvements compared with another group who were not sent any healing. The group sent distant healing needed less medication, had less heart failure and had much lower incidence of complications than the other group. It didn't matter what the relationship was between the background religion or beliefs the healers sending the thoughts had and those of the group of patients. Quite simply, when the healers sent out healing thoughts the receivers benefited.

In another experiment, at the Sierra Health Institute in California, a group of people were sent distant healing by two healers 200 miles away. Again none of the recipients knew that this was being done, and electromyographic (EMG) recording machines were attached to the patients. These machines measure how much electromagnetic radiation is coming from the muscles and show what the nervous system is doing – how relaxed or tense the body is. In the people sent distant healing the muscle recordings in the chest and lower back showed huge changes – a great reduction in tension and increase in relaxation. Just what we want in our horses.

In 1998, other US researchers, this time at Duke University, noted that patients who were prayed for (i.e. sent distant healing) recovered 50 to 100 per cent better than a group who were not. The senders of the healing came from a wide range of people from around the world, and all had different beliefs and ways of sending the healing thoughts. It just demonstrates how powerful healing intent and thought is.

By distant healing producing this effect it can be seen how horses can benefit as well. We can link with horses we've lost contact with, or who are away from us for some reason or even horses we've never met. I often send out distant healing to all the thousands of horses around the world who are in terrible distress, fear and pain. We don't need to know where the horses are or who they are as the healing will reach those who need it. By this method all of us can help those horses and give some comfort. I have often sent distant healing to horses for clients who have contacted me and whose animals I have not been able to see because they lived too far away from me and have had very good responses. Several case studies are included in Chapter 5 for further reading.

Can anyone give healing?

Quite simply the opportunity is there for everyone to tune in to healing energies as long as the person giving the healing wants to help. There needs be an overwhelming urge to be a healing person not a hurting person. We may hurt the horse unintentionally – emotionally and mentally – by ignoring or misunderstanding problems that it tries to communicate to us. This stress can then affect the horse's physical health.

By attuning to the healing energies we open up a higher channel of communication, which should help us to understand the vital information from the horse – and help to prevent us from hurting.

To want to touch or send thoughts to a sick or troubled horse (indeed any person or animal) is the most natural thing in the world. That is the basic instinct which healers then go on to develop, further channelling energy from a powerful, divine, universal source to the horse that is in need. Healing is done through love and that is the most important requirement needed by the healer – unselfish love offering a helping hand. Because it is done through love it is safe for any horse and also the person giving the healing. However, the guidelines in this book are intended for use on your own horse or pony only and would not to be sufficient to enable you to practise as a professional healer. Nor would they allow you to join a recognised healing association as a member.

Healing can be given for any condition, and can be used to target specific areas such as a wound or can be given generally to help the horse anywhere that it may be needed. Everyone has different strengths and weaknesses and some people will be able to develop greater sensitivity in channelling healing than others. They will be more 'in tune' with their horses or may find it easier to work with one horse than another. Healing is still effective on some level even if the giver is unable to 'feel' anything and so it is still well worth practising for the benefit of your horse.

Are there times when healing should not be given?

There are some times when it is not advisable to give healing to horses and during these times it is a good idea to have healing ourselves from a professional healer who has developed strong abilities.

If we are very ill or going through some sort of major problem or crisis in life, for example, it not advisable to attempt to give healing. Animals are very sensitive to energy and at these times we will be depleted so the horse will be resistant to what we are trying to achieve. It is better on these occasions to ask someone else who is better balanced emotionally and physically to give healing to the horse. Chapter 6 gives further details on this subject.

Knowledge and learning increase our power as healers for they help our brain to focus healing intent into the horse's body and mind. The more anatomical understanding we have, and the more knowledge of the horse's natural needs and reasons why it could be unhappy, the stronger the healing will become.

Healing as a gift

People often say to me, 'Ah, but healing is a gift, isn't it? I couldn't do it.' Well, yes and no. Every person may give healing – it is the most natural thing in the world to lay the hands on the sick and needy. However, some people are gifted healers in the same way that some people are gifted musicians, artists or singers. Being gifted is an extra depth and dimension, something that people appear to be born with.

Until we try, though, we don't know how gifted we are as healers and like anything else in life the power and strength doesn't come overnight – it requires practice, patience and dedication to achieve. There are different levels of awareness and sensitivity, and to explore the gift a healer needs to spend a long time developing natural abilities.

Intuitive healing

Some healers are intuitive or clairvoyant (which means to see clearly), and this extra-sensory attunement is something that falls into the category of being gifted. Today, though, mankind has hurtled away from a rapport

WHAT IS HEALING FOR HORSES?

with each other, with animals and with nature. That rapport enhances intuitive skills. Thankfully, there is a growing interest in understanding our spiritual side and regaining lost natural abilities. Also a desire to return to getting in touch with all our senses, thereby increasing our awareness of the meaning of life.

As a child I began to demonstrate extra-sensory gifts and these now mean that I am an animal communicator – able to see or pick up information from auras, energy fields and through my fingertips by touching a horse. This information is never a diagnosis, as only a veterinary surgeon may do that, but an awareness of energy blockage in certain areas. Sometimes I ask a client to call in a vet for a seemingly healthy horse because I am concerned about an area of blocked energy, which may indicate a problem. Some vets have asked me to visit a horse to help pinpoint the area of pain or energy blockage, or why a horse is emotionally disturbed. I am able to pick up images and information from the horse's past which can explain behavioural disturbances. This ability to tune in to the horse also helps me to target the vital force more specifically with my healing. It makes the healing process more active and powerful. Usually it is through the same universal energies from which the healing comes that I tune in to receive information about the horse. This comes in the form of words or pictures, but sometimes the information comes directly from the horse in the form of a mental conversation.

The ability to be a visionary or intuitive healer is a gift, but many people have these qualities and don't develop them or they push them to one side. People talk about having 'hunches' or 'feelings' about things – well, that's a start. When you give healing to your horse have an open mind and just see what you feel with your hands, with your mind, with your heart. Set aside regular healing time and begin a journey of your spiritual development as you set out to help your horse. It may take a long time; my own healer training with a recognised organisation was three years, and it took many more years to build up to the strength that I have now. However, the sacrifices and study have been worth it and it has really enriched my life, enabling me to help a lot of horses and therefore a lot of people too.

Many years ago when I was developing my clairvoyant ability I decided that I would use it to help my healing to be more profound, and not for trivial or superficial reasons. I wanted only to use my extra-sensory vision for healing work relevant to the welfare of animals or people. I cannot therefore tell someone whether a horse prefers his blue rug or his pink one but I can tell them where he hurts physically and what happened years ago so that he hurts emotionally. It is with this knowledge that I focus into the energy field of the horse's body to heal him on all levels. Neither do I use my gifts to make predictions. Clients sometimes ask me if I can 'see' whether the horse or pony will win this or that competition or be suitable for what they want it to do. I answer that I cannot because that is not important to the horse and irrelevant in terms of healing.

Does healing need a faith to be effective?

Healing is non-denominational and no particular faiths or beliefs are necessary and, anyway, there isn't a horse born yet who has a religious faith or any concept of religion. The horse simply understands and relates to the forces of nature and the universe and the natural order of life. Hands-on healing is the most natural therapy in the world and therefore something the horse readily accepts.

When I have been giving healing to a human I have asked them to have an openness and a trust in the fact that I am trying to help them. When giving healing to horses I have found that the openness to accept the healing is already and naturally there although the trust may not be. If the horse is distrustful, however, this appears not to matter as the healing is accepted on a much deeper level than this initial emotion. Horses seem to be ready to accept inner change and possess the motivation to let that change improve their lives if possible. Only on a handful of occasions over the years have I come across a horse who did not accept healing at some level.

Religions have frequently closely guarded the secrets of the invisible healing energies of the universe and other organisations have come along the way to repackage healing as a new discovery although it has always been literally at everyone's fingertips. I have beliefs and my faith is very strong but I do not belong to a particular group nor attend a church. I have friends from a wide range of cultures, nationalities and religious backgrounds and we spend many a happy hour sharing opinions and views. We all appear to have an inkling of the truth of creation and the meaning of life and there are many similarities in our beliefs. I believe that life isn't just a random soup of interactive energies, but that there is a divine source that it all relates to and which controls it. Every religion has tried to interpret it and there have been many prophets, but it is my belief also that human understanding is limited at present so our interpretation becomes distorted. I respect, however, that everyone makes their own journey in their own way to understand the source of this spiritual nature, with each person having individual beliefs to find a meaningful way of life.

I have many times experienced a great supernatural power and have had some very unusual experiences – it is this power which I call God. I see God as an overall and infinite intelligence, which is the source of healing. It is always there for us to tap into as we do when we give healing treatments and which, as I have explained earlier in the book, is more than an adjustment of energy. Where the source is actually situated is the mystery to which mankind continually strives to seek the answer. The healer uses his or her own electromagnetic field to channel energy to the horse, but it is not the healer's own energy that actually does the healing. That is drawn from the source of all life mysteriously situated somewhere in the universe.

Although I believe that I am channelling healing from God you can believe that you are channelling healing from anywhere – the sun, the moon or the stars, for example – and the energy source is the same. An important thing to remember is that you can't just force healing on to any person or any animal – you need to have permission from the horse for the healing to be accepted and the horse will judge you by what is in your heart. Healing should be offered to the horse with love. The most important thing for someone to believe when they give healing is that they are going to help. It is the intent to heal which the healer must have in his or her heart. The intent becomes in itself a very powerful source of energy linking to the horse. Attuning to the healing energy requires a mixture of empathy, compassion and intent and the more strongly we can direct these feelings to the horse the stronger the healing will be. We need to remember that the horse, like the human, will have a need for healing on three levels – emotional, mental and physical.

When healing does not mean recovery

The one thing that is guaranteed for every living creature, including plants and trees, is that there will be an end to the life on this earth. As with us, our horse, when it is born, immediately starts the process and pathway towards death – the end of the physical life. It is inevitable, either due to the ageing process when nothing works very well any more or earlier, due to disease or injury. After an illness or injury the horse may not recover the same level of previous health but healing aims to strengthen the process to the best possible level. As healing is effective on an emotional as well as a physical level it can give a feeling of inner peace and calmness, and also helps release pent-up energy due to the stresses surrounding orthodox treatment and recovery.

When cells in the horse's body are too badly diseased or damaged for the horse's own inner processes to be stimulated into recovery by healing, then death may result. When I have treated terminally ill horses just before death, owners have reported an air of peace with the horse, which has helped the owners too at this very traumatic time. With these horses there have sometimes been dramatic but temporary improvements after healing (the horse has felt energised and feels at peace), but I always add a word of caution to the owners about this. It is simply not possible for healing to repair severely damaged or diseased body parts and in those cases healing is aimed at giving a feeling of peace and calmness to the horse in the last stages of the physical life.

We are on a journey that has many stages and release of the physical body is one of those stages. There eventually comes a time for the horse to leave the physical body and for its life force to move on to a higher level. We call that process death but it is, in fact, the releasing of the life force or essence. Healing cannot stop that happening but it can help to make the transition a positive process for both horse and human.

In today's world where science has created so many 'quick fixes' and living for here and now is mostly the norm, many societies don't accept death very well any more. We see it as not natural yet it is actually the most natural thing in our lives because it is the one thing that can be guaranteed. The hardest part is coping with the physical end of a young horse who had so much promise and was so full of life until things went wrong, or dealing with the demise of a horse who met a sudden and violent end. At these times owners may also benefit from healing treatment. It can bring much comfort and a sense that the horse is indeed linking back deep into our own soul. Our shared energy continues and lives on through eternity.

3
Why horses need healing

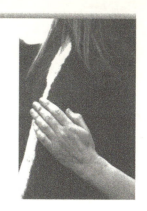

*'Spirit to Spirit,
I will reach out
recognising you as part of myself,
and myself as part of you.'*
            Margrit Coates

EVERYTHING IN NATURE, including the horse, consists of a complex system of rhythms and energies. Each cell and each organ in the horse has its own cycle and set of rhythms, which are influenced by the horse's energy field, the fields of the earth and the energies of people relating to the horse. Horses need healing for a great many reasons, not least the fact that their natural lifestyle has been disturbed, and many of them have a life of severe restriction with owners who are oblivious to their cries for help and to their pain. We have all made mistakes with our horses and I'd be the first to step forward and raise my hand in admission, but we do the best we can with the knowledge and information that we have at the time. As we evolve, we see there is a better way for the relationship as a whole. Until fairly recently very little research had been done into why a horse does what it does or into its mind – even less has been researched into the horse's emotions, and this is where hands-on healing can play such an important role.

There is a culture clash between the horse and the human: both cultures are wildly different. In its natural environment a horse will walk and graze for up to 16 hours a day and will have friends and a social structure, relying on its finely tuned instincts to survive. Buried deep in the genes of the horse lies the basis for its survival and very little has changed for the horse over the years in this respect. The horse is in tune with the weather, the stars, the tides, and the seasons and his mind has the ability to interact with the earth's electromagnetic fields, something that most humans have lost the knack of. Things are beginning to change, thankfully, and more and more people seek to explore their spiritual roots and to include their horses in that experience for we are linked to them and our journey in life includes walking by their side. Healing plays a vital and fundamental role in that journey and gives both horse and owner a deeper foundation, a more fruitful bond, which switches on a light in the world where the horse's pleas created a darkness. After healing, owners frequently report that their horses appear to be happier and show more personality – their sensory inputs appear to be better co-ordinated by the network of neurons in the brain.

There is a growth of professionals, including vets, trainers, riders, and managers, who are encouraging a holistic approach and throwing into question how we view the equestrian philosophy. The time is right for improvement and change because people are looking for a better understanding of their own lives and a return to more natural methods of healthcare and management of the environment. Everything around us, all living things, including our horses, are part of our world so to understand our lives better we need to become closer to our animals too. This is something that people frequently say to me: healing opens up a better understanding, a stronger bond between them and their horse. Healing is as natural as the horse and healing enriches the lives of everyone who experiences it. Often people find it difficult to describe in words because it is such a subtle and deep feeling, which helps them to take a step further forwards in both spiritual enlightenment and understanding their horse.

Mankind has been domesticating the horse for over 6000 years but it hasn't evolved very much in that time to be anything other than an animal in tune with his natural instincts and his species group. Nothing has changed in the nature of the horse and after all this time and involvement with mankind there isn't a foal born who doesn't have to be trained to be ridden or perform in some way, which is when the problems begin. The horse's responses are still finely attuned to the wild and it is to the horse's credit and honesty that he allows himself to submit to the human will, and why he is so often misunderstood. From this breakdown in communication comes a great deal of the breakdown in the horse's energy field and resulting chaos in energy patterns. It is one of the fundamental reasons why horses need healing. Another is the fact that the horse is now wholly dependent on the human race for its survival and needs and is usually viewed as a working animal.

Let us be horse healers

- ❖ Healing is a foundation for physical, mental and emotional repair of the horse. It is one of the tools of the holistic approach.
- ❖ All physiological conditions result from disharmony in energy patterns, which may include, even partly, the emotions.
- ❖ We must understand and keep in the forefront of the mind the purpose of our true spiritual relationship with the horse.
- ❖ We also need to be aware of how horses respond to healing and be prepared to give healing at any time.
- ❖ Keep yourself in good emotional, physical and mental health. This in turn helps to keep the horse balanced.

As we go about our business and our pleasure, let us hear our conscience and not forget the horse we are responsible for – who so depends on our charity and goodwill for health and freedom. Let us be horse healers.

Look at the complete picture

Horses submit to the will of humans and a horse with a good owner and/or rider will submit through respect and trust, but the unfortunate horse in a bad home will submit through fear and hatred. These are the screaming horses, the horses that leave a dark echo in the world from their inner turmoil and pain. I treat many horses whose lives have been blighted in this way and these are the lucky ones with new owners who realise that healing can help them to really let go of the past, which also affects the present and the future. Too often we forget the horse is an individual with its own capabilities and limits. Not all can fit the ideal picture of a perfect trot, a perfect outline and jumping high fences. Owners and riders frequently push average ability horses and ponies beyond their comfort zone and capabilities, causing severe physical, mental and emotional stress. I often see these unfortunate animals for healing treatments, which helps to take away a great deal of the inner anguish caused by being asked to do too much. We are not all marathon runners, great athletes, gymnasts or supreme intellectuals and neither are all equines. A happier horse is one whose owner recognises who that horse person is and what he or she can truly do. Owners have reported that sharing healing with their horses builds up a deeper understanding of their partner and who that horse is.

Horses can be unsettled for many years and owners can get to their wits' end trying to sort out first one problem then another, seeking symptomatic treatment when the root cause is much deeper. Healing treats the horse holistically, aiming for balance which if necessary other practitioners can also build on. When we give healing to the horse we receive a subtle expansion of our own understanding and in turn we receive healing as the universal energy embraces us.

All horses need healing at some time or other because they cannot express themselves or communicate with words. As a result, a large and frequent amount of misunderstanding takes place between horse and human, which creates an imbalance in the energy field. Even a horse from a good home who is trying to communicate a problem that goes unheard or unheeded will become disturbed in some way as the stress knocks the energy field out of balance. Sometimes it's small and minor, sometimes dramatic and major, and these horses may become more prone to injury or illness, or may start to exhibit problems in their work. If we get into the habit

Imagine the cosmic noise and the darkness from thousands of horses silently screaming, 'Help me please and heal me.'

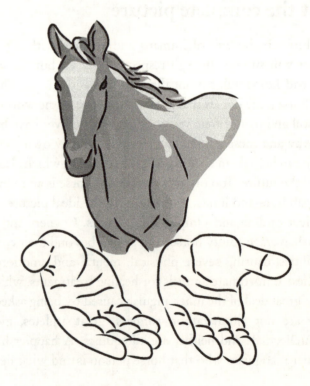

of healing and opening up the intensive lines of communication that healing develops through our touch and into our minds we should begin to get more from the horse and, of course, then enjoy our time and relationship with them much better. Imagine what a nightmare it would be to be taken to live with another species who spoke a foreign language and who didn't understand our language at all. Imagine the horror of shouting, 'Please don't make me run around for I've got a terrible headache.' 'I'm bored and lonely, get me out of here.' 'Help me, my back hurts.' 'I miss my family and friends.' In reply to our pleas and requests our keepers then punish us and hurt us so that in the end we become depressed and depleted.

The horse's emotions

I was lecturing to a group of people from a riding club on healing for horses when one of the questions asked was to expand on my belief that horses had emotions like humans do. Horses have emotions without a doubt, maybe on a different level to humans but the type of emotions are the same and relevant to their species, and how they communicate and behave. I asked this group to give me a list of human emotions, and they called out, 'Love, fear, hatred, anger, grief, resentment, jealousy, worry.' I then asked which of these emotions applied to humans only and not to horses. The room fell silent and no one replied. Emotions are not exclusive to humans and it is arrogant to think so. Horses have emotions and when they are denied the free expression of them or express negative emotions due to poor management, problems frequently occur, which we then often blame the horse for.

It always upsets me to feel a rush of emotion come away from a horse during healing, something pent up and eating away inside. Sometimes the owner feels these emotions come away too and on those occasions is usually moved to tears, as the horse's emotional pain hits them in the heart or solar plexus. When I have treated abused and ill-treated horses at rescue centres their terrible emotional turmoil has left me tearful and drained for a couple of days afterwards. An important point to note here is that if any horse is troubled then that will affect us too as all energy is shared to some extent. It is another very good reason to give healing to horses to help keep everything in balance, and certainly vets recognise that depressed and emotionally troubled horses are less able to recover from health problems.

Emotions are feelings and thoughts and these vibrations from the horse's brain and heart travel through all of its systems, including the blood stream, nerve endings and muscles. So the thought process of the horse is important and relevant to healing. If the horse is sad, depressed, lonely, angry, worried, confused, cold, hurting, then those thoughts will trigger a certain oscillation or frequency of energy which in turn will travel throughout the horse's whole body. This imbalance affects all the other energy levels in all of the systems and organs and begins to be destructive. In my experience, this chaotic energy can remain for many years, leading to all sorts of problems, and healing can be very effective in re-establishing the status quo. Frequently, many of the horse's problems can improve or even disappear.

A horse is a person who looks like a horse. It is made of blood, flesh, bone and nerve endings just like we are. The big difference is that we can express our fears and frustrations and have a good cry if need be but horses cannot. That energy turmoil of emotion goes round and round inside, and healing aims to free the horse from it.

The eye to the soul

When I look into a horse's eye I sense infinite space and such powerful intuition and spiritual awareness. When you give healing to your horse, as it relaxes and trusts what you are doing, stand by the head with your hand on the neck and look into that eye. You will see what I mean. Spirit is being revealed through the eye of the horse and received by the eye of the human. Sometimes this eye contact is so powerful and strong that for a second you may feel as though an old soul is looking back at you. And so it is – the old soul that communicates through your healing touch and belongs to thousands of years of the horse's ancestors and history. Love, dependency, independency, all communicated in a split second through the healing touch and intent.

Have you ever found yourself, looking into the horse's eye, feeling suddenly disconcerted or very emotional? It is because at that very moment your own soul recognised the soul of the horse as being part of your spiritual family. When a horse looks me in the eye I can frequently hear words quite clearly – a message from that horse – sometimes funny, sometimes poignant, sometimes profound. Often when I am giving healing and standing close to the horse's head there is such a power and

WHY HORSES NEED HEALING

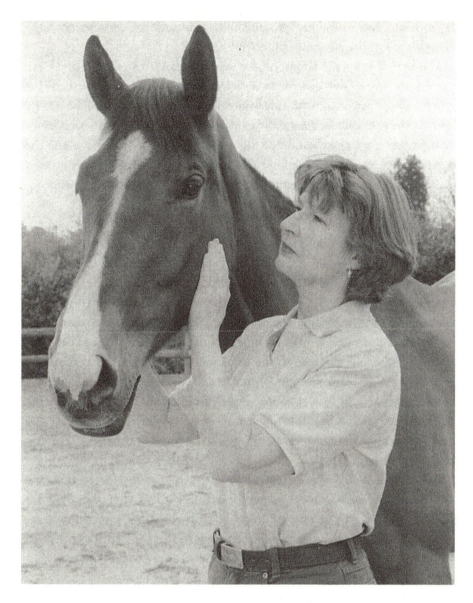

During healing there is an intensification of electromagnetic radiation from the horse's eye, stimulated by the healer's touch. It is through the horse's eye that we can sense its soul.

intensity that draws me into the eye that a thousand words pass between me and the horse in a fraction of a second. And yet there are no words that I can use to adequately describe that moment or the spiritual knowledge imparted.

I am aware that not everyone believes that a horse has a soul – a link through the life force to the universal God – but I feel that denying that they do gives mankind an excuse for lack of respect. It allows the belief that there is no accountability for selfishness and lack of conscience. Such thoughts are not at all compatible with healing.

The horse's eye is the largest of any mammal that lives on earth and has a magical and expressive quality to it. Scientific research has confirmed that eyes transmit electromagnetic radiation, one of the components of the energy field. When you start linking with your horse with healing you will notice a 'charging up' or intensification of this radiation between your eye and the horse's eye. It may happen only briefly to begin with but as you progress in healing confidence, these periods should increase in length and intensity.

Communicating with the horse on a spiritual level

With practice, healers can feel with their fingertips on the horse vibratory information that precisely specifies the activities which are taking place within the horse's body. Some of these activities are on a physical plane but some are from the life force or essence of the horse – its spirit. It is unique to that horse and with practice and sensitivity it is possible to distinguish the feel of the spiritual energy from the whole. It is during those moments that we really feel we 'know' the horse and can often receive messages from its mind through thought – often as a flash of insight. It is a two-way communication and it is at those special times, when we feel the horse's spiritual energy, that the horse feels our own. I've seen many people hug their horses after healing and say things like, 'I didn't know that's how you felt,' or 'If only I'd known.'

It is a time to offer our deepest love and to ask for forgiveness and understanding, for help to know what the horse truly needs and to ask for the healing power to grow ever stronger in us. It is a very moving, humbling and thought-provoking experience to realise the depth of spiritual communication that healing can open up between us and our horse.

Insufficient daylight

Daylight is essential for a horse's optimum health and a fully balanced energy field. Sunlight plays a vital role in vitamin D production and bone formation, thus helping bones to be strong. The sun's rays have also been shown to have an effect on blood pressure and the digestive system and help the natural body clock to maintain its balance, and there are many other bodily processes in which daylight has a role. The pineal gland in the brain monitors the amount of daylight it receives and is the site of influence of the biological time clock, monitoring the horse's lifestyle from birth to death, by way of hormone secretions into the bloodstream. If the pineal does not function fully and the energy balance around that gland is depleted then other glands in the body will be affected and the failure of any of them will cause serious illness – behaviour can also be affected as well. A horse may have energy blockages in any of the glands relating to the endocrine system if it has been kept inside for long periods and healing can play a role in helping to rebalance and revitalise these areas.

Horses, like humans, can be affected by SAD – Seasonal Affective Disorder – and it is thought that lack of sunlight through the eyes is a critical factor in this debilitating condition. Daylight is also essential for hormonal function, which is why brood mares can be brought into season artificially by the use of daylight lamps in stables. There is a direct link between the daylight from the universe and the horse because one of the levels of the energy field is a light wave, so lack of light from insufficient daylight affects the whole health balance. It is one of the reasons why it is depressing for the horse to be in gloomy and dark conditions for much of its time, and riders and owners will probably not be getting the best from

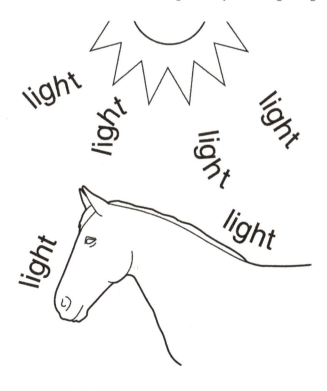

Horses need some free time in daylight every day for optimum health and a fully balanced energy field. If your horse is confined because of veterinary treatment/instruction, see if you can use a stable where the horse can put its head over the door into good bright light and use a light, airy stable. Check with your vet in case of contraindications.

Warning

Horses who are turned out do need shade that they can rest in if they need to. Shade may be provided either by trees and bushes or a field shelter. Check with your vet about outdoor time and exposure to sunlight for horses with liver problems as serious photosensitisation can result. Follow veterinary advice on restricted turnout for sick and injured horses and those with sweet itch.

the horse. Research with animals has shown that illness is associated with less light being emitted from the body's meridians and it can be a contributing factor in equine problems. Certainly during healing I have often noticed a depletion of energy over meridians and chakras of over-stabled horses. Fly fringes, ear covers, herbal lotions, field shelters and free access to stables are by far the best solutions to avoiding the nuisance of flies as opposed to locking the horse up for long periods. If stabling horses during the day is unavoidable they will enjoy being turned out as early as possible in the afternoon to benefit from the light. I find in general when I am giving healing that the energy field of horses who have good access to daylight vibrates on a higher plane than horses who spend a lot of time inside. Sunshine, of course, has a feel good factor, which is going to help us get the best from our horses too, and is healing in itself.

The confined horse

Horses in the natural state spend many hours in the day grazing and moving about. When they are prevented from taking part in these activities, stereotypic behaviour can manifest itself. Crib biting, weaving and wind sucking are human-created conditions to relieve stress and boredom. These are all actions that the over-stabled and misunderstood horse displays and which he frequently gets further punished for with cruel devices applied to prevent these 'vices' and which make the horse's distress even worse because he then has no way to alleviate the terrible stress. These are not 'vices' but signs of depression and severe unhappiness and the actions the horse performs releases a chemical called enkephalin, which in all animals helps to relieve distress and has a painkilling effect. So we can see how cruel it is to stop the horse when it is his only way of trying to keep sane.

WHY HORSES NEED HEALING

Horses, particularly youngsters, need to lie down, and roll. Watching ponies in the New Forest, where I live, shows how much time they spend doing this and how much pleasure they get from it. Over-stabled horses are frequently denied this pleasure or get 'cast' after lying down in a restricted space, causing further stress and injury. Interestingly, at the end of a healing session this type of horse often reacts as though waking from a good sleep, stretching, arching the neck and relaxing each hind leg out in turn as if demonstrating how the healing has offered them an experience of peace normally denied.

A client who watched me give healing to a young horse recently commented afterwards it was 'as though he is just waking from a big sleep'. Sometimes this reaction comes from a horse with lots of current freedom but who was denied the opportunity to lie down as a youngster. When giving healing to these horses I have found their energy very blocked and sluggish. They have responded well to treatment, however, and become much more relaxed and at peace with the world. Sleep and rest is nature's time when the body tries to repair and heal itself, and very stressed and over-stabled horses do not rest properly, thereby being deprived even more of good mental and physical health. Because it is so deeply relaxing, healing offers the horse a kind of 'mini-sleep', thus helping the disturbed energy field around the systems to recover.

The palpable sadness that pervades from horses for kept too long 'in prison' hangs heavy in the aura of the world and it affects the people who

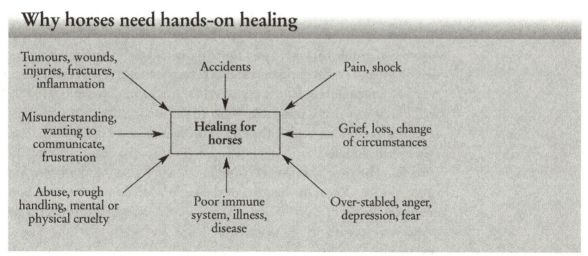

Why horses need hands-on healing

Signs of being too confined

Research into horses who are stabled for long periods has shown that biochemical changes similar to those that occur in human prison inmates takes place, leading to behavioural changes. Studies on prisoners who have been confined for a long time demonstrates that these people show the following traits in an attempt to alleviate boredom, depression and stress:

- **Increased aggression and violence to others.**
- **Displays of self-mutilation.**
- **Repetitive and compulsive behaviour.**

handle them and blights their own aura too. Part of living a healing life is establishing our own inner peace and to be fair and honest we need to offer conditions to the horse which help it find peace too.

As well as cooping horses up in stables for long periods we then barge in to this small space of theirs and do things to them, which can stress these horses even more until they become aggressive towards us or turn their backs on us. They are frequently chastised for this behaviour, which just makes them even more anxious and in turmoil. We can see what this distress is doing to the horse's energy field and the chaos that can result, and where healing is going to play a vital role to rebalance that energy. However, if the reasons the horse is displaying signs of severe stress aren't addressed, then the healing benefits may not hold for more than a few days.

One such horse I was asked to give healing to was a large cob mare with severe skin problems. I was upset to see the mare kept in a narrow stall and tied by a chain with a chock at the end (a heavy weight) – a very outdated way of keeping horses. The horse couldn't turn or lie down and faced the wall during her many miserable hours in the gloom. The mare was very responsive to healing and at the end of the session most of the lumps and bumps had smoothed on the horse's skin as she was so deeply relaxed and peaceful. The owner, however, wouldn't hear of keeping the horse any other way, so I knew the benefits of the healing would not last long. Sure enough a couple of days later the horse's skin was as bad as ever and the owner was looking to homeopathy to 'cure' her, when what she needed was freedom and fresh air.

Unnatural food

I pick up many levels of unbalanced energy when I give healing to horses and often there is a problem in the intestinal area. Horses are designed to graze over long periods and research is now also showing increasing evidence that feeding horses high levels of concentrates and stabling them for long periods can be very harmful in that it adversely affects the level of serotonin found in the brain and intestines. Serotonin is produced by the brain stem and acts as a neurotransmitter and vasoconstrictor. Low levels of this essential chemical lead to depression and displays of stressed behaviour so we come back to the fact that the best life for a horse is one which is as natural as possible, and which becomes a 'healing life'. It is better for us in the long run as well.

It is highly possible that the constant stress produced in horses by long confinements and unnatural feeds is causing them to have delicate stomachs. Horses that roam pastures eat a lot of roughage and a good deal of low-quality food. They also eat often, not going for long periods without food, which over-stabled horses are forced to do. A study in Germany of more than 1000 cases of colic showed that the highest incidences were associated with weather changes, which would not upset a free-roaming horse, used to the nature's elements. Vets in the US have also noticed that foals that are suddenly confined in stables can become so distressed that perforating ulcers can result in death. When there is an imbalance in the digestive areas I notice that during healing there can be a lot of gurgling and release of wind, as the energies begin to flow and change.

Insufficient water

Water within the horse plays a major role in detecting vibratory information in its body and is one of the ways the horse is helped to keep healthy. It is a fact also taken advantage of by homeopathic vets, who use the memory storage of water in conjunction with remedies. Before I studied complementary medicine I wondered why some horses had a very heavy and flat feel to their energies. But with experience I noticed that these horses usually had either very little water in the field or stable or dirty and dusty water – they weren't drinking enough for optimum health. When water changes were made and I returned a week or so later there was a noticeable improvement in the speed of pulsing and energy flow that I could detect through my fingertips. It is vitally important for long-term health and a balanced energy field that horses have access to fresh, clean water at all times.

Early weaning

Early weaning and sudden weaning can also result in stereotypic patterns of behaviour or 'vices', as research undertaken by vets in the UK has shown. All too often I pick up in a horse emotional disturbance, shock and grief related to weaning. Later in life this early trauma can lead to all sorts of general health conditions as well as behavioural problems, which can affect the horse's useful life. Sadly sometimes these horses can become too unstable to ride or handle and even healing has not been able to help some of the very traumatised cases that I have come across where the problems were too deeply entrenched in the horse. Weaning is often a commercially based decision but perhaps a better time to do this is around 12 months when a foal would wean naturally in the wild, and there are kind and beneficial ways, which holistic vets and natural trainers can advise on.

We need to remember that a foal is a child and it is our responsibility to offer it as good a start possible for its future in this world. It is a good idea if someone has acquired a young horse that has been weaned early and/or traumatically to ask an animal healer to help rebalance the emotional field. It is also important for healing to be offered to an older horse that has an early weaning background. I have come across lots of health problems in these horses, including skin conditions, sarcoids and depressed immune systems. The necessity for healing for foals begins very early in their lives and I advocate healing for them as soon as possible to help realise their full potential. Foals will be sensitive to signals from the energy field of the mare and other horses nearby, and if there is a problem of any sort the foal will be affected by it.

Lack of company

Horses naturally like to be touched and in the wild will spend hours grooming each other. Horses form special friendships and will groom with those horses more than others. Sometimes a person has said to me that they have separated horses because they bonded too strongly with one another, which I find very sad and unnecessary. More enlightened people can make use of this natural need. For example, some competition horses travel with stable companions to help them settle in a strange yard.

When we touch a horse we are contacting every part of its physical body and mind through the living matrix, a field of interactive energy linking every part with each other. When horses touch each other they are communicating through the living matrix and it is a form of healing that they also give each other, as therapeutic as humans holding hands. It is something we should not deny them for doing so denies them the healing touch from their own kind. When we touch a horse we increase the flow of shared energy and this touch may be from our hands or from our bodies. When they lay their hands on to a horse, healers are deliberately increasing the flow of beneficial shared energy. We can transmit to the horse a feeling of balanced or disturbed energy through our bodies and it is something we should be aware of when riding rather than always being too ready to blame the horse for having an off day, if things are less than

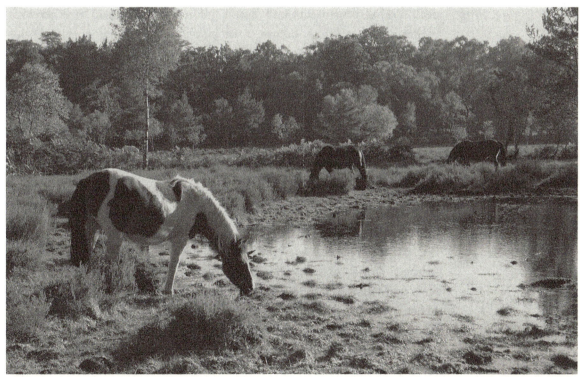

A group of horses in a natural environment: open spaces to move and graze freely, plenty of natural shade, and fresh water from a stream.

'Vices' and problems can be caused by human intervention of the horse's natural needs

- Lack of company.
- Too much time inside a stable.
- A stressful routine.
- Aggressive and/or impatient handling.
- Work that is beyond the capabilities of that particular horse.
- Impatient/inconsiderate instruction or schooling, the horse not understanding or being rushed.
- Early weaning.

Healing plays an important role in releasing and rebalancing the negative energy that results from these problems and offers the horse inner peace and an improved sense of wellbeing.

ideal. It is for this reason that I always link horse and human together with my healing for it is no good just treating the horse if the owner is badly out of balance. It is often a shared 'letting go' during healing that enables both horse and human to proceed forward in their relationship.

In our attempts to domesticate the horse we have often deprived it of its ability to communicate with other horses. Imagine how frustrating it would be if we couldn't express our personality with other humans, talk to them, socialise with friends, just be a human being. In depriving horses of the chance to talk to each other in a relaxed and free manner we create a breakdown of inner harmony. I often find healing going in to a very deep inner core in horses to clear emotional disturbance due to lack of opportunity for full natural expression.

I recently treated a horse, now very luckily in a wonderful home. He had been hunted extensively as a two-year-old, having been weaned suddenly and far too early, so he'd had big shocks in his early life, physically, mentally and emotionally. This horse quickly became very sleepy during the healing and relaxed deeply, showing big changes in respiratory rhythm. I had my hands on the horse's neck and back and could feel that inside this horse there were many tears. Suddenly I was aware of a wave of energy pulsating through his body from the heart chakra along to the dural membrane (which runs through the spine). A split second later the horse arched his back and let out a piercing scream. Then his body deflated and he stood with his head hanging low, swaying gently, looking drained but very peaceful.

I was shocked, the horse had screamed, and I could see it had shocked the people who were watching too. In those few seconds that scream had communicated all the fear, anger, pain and sadness that the horse had bottled up over the years. It had a profound effect on me and gave me a lot to think about, as it was the first time that it had happened during one of my treatments. Sighing, grunting, yawning, licking and chewing I was used to when a horse let go emotionally, but screaming showed just how bad the inner turmoil could get and how it could be bottled up. Six hours later his owner told me the horse was showing signs of several changes already, he was calmer, more friendly and more 'talkative'. Without the healing that scream would have continued to exist inside the horse, creating more energy imbalance and turmoil, and potentially leading to all sorts of future problems.

A deprived and unfulfilled horse can eventually become an injury or illness prone horse. When a horse communicates with another horse it's not just an emotional response but a release of physical energies as he flicks his ears, curls his lips, kicks out, chases, grunts, squeals, nods and runs around and then relaxes. Because humans don't display any of these characteristics we often worry about them in the horse and stop them from displaying these natural releases of energy by separating them or punishing them. We often don't allow horses to socialise because we don't understand their needs and worry that they may hurt each other. It is always a possibility, but the more horses go out regularly in groups where they can form friendships the less there seems to be a problem. The world's greatest horsemen and women recognise this and work their horses from a very natural lifestyle.

Information from the horse

We need the horse to submit to us out of respect and trust not fear and hatred. Healing helps us to build that communication. It is the natural link, the natural communication between the horse and the human, a journey between the spirit of the horse and the spirit of the healer. It is giving and receiving at the highest level.

There is a co-operation between horse and rider with both parties giving different things in the way of commitment. The horse submits to work that the human requires it to do with little idea of its own physical strength, and the human will give a great deal of time and money in pursuing the horse–human relationship. The relationship works or not depending on the level of communication between them, and receiving communication from the horse is part of the 'healing soup', which transmits not through words but on a much higher level. The information we receive in this way is instantaneous and comes in on several planes all at once – intuitive, emotional, physical. We 'know' what we have received but then we have to put that into words. Sometimes there is a delayed reaction and it takes a couple of minutes to translate the communication, to vocalise it.

When I first began to give healing to horses I found it quite difficult sometimes to put into words the feelings that the horse communicated to me. But as time went on it became easier to explain, and now I often get a physical sensation as well, particularly if the horse has pain somewhere. Information is transferred from sender (healer) to receiver (horse) and then decoded, and, of course, it works both ways. A horse receives information from people and in its own way, at its own level of understanding, decodes this information. The horse is a very sensitive and highly tuned animal and this is why healing is helpful, necessary even, when there has been an overload of unbalancing information for the horse.

How do horses communicate with us? Thoughts and feelings vibrate with energy and it is that vibration that we pick up on and register – the art is understanding and interpreting the vibrations. Humans have sophisticated thinking which enables them to tap into thoughts on an energy level, but so do horses on their own level. It is this energy level that also associates with healing energy, and we are back to understanding that everything is interrelated, everything is part of the whole, which affects each level of healing energy.

We can now see the complex nature of the horse's energy field on all levels of communication and where healing can play a role in releasing pent-up emotion for the frustrated horse offering some peace of mind, soul and body. The horse does not live according to human values, just as the human does not live according to horse values, but the emotions both species display are similar, albeit on a different level. It is not recognising this that can cause horses so much anguish and distress and why I am often requested to help them with healing.

Expecting too much of a horse

Natural trainers such as Monty Roberts have done a great deal to further the welfare of the horse by introducing to modern society natural methods of horsemanship, which try to avoid negative confrontation and bad behaviour from the trainer. It is a big step forwards for the benefit of the horse, but we're not quite there yet. Horses and riders will always have falls and accidents, and there will always sadly be people who choose to be hurters rather than healers (maybe even unwittingly). But knowing who the horse truly is and understanding the species will help us to enjoy them more and get more out of the relationship. It is a time for the ego to take a back seat, a good thing for our spiritual development generally. Riding with healing flowing through our hands and bodies will lead to a better rapport and increased sensitivity, for healing hands are giving hands in more ways than one.

An important area where we may stress the horse unduly if we are not careful is in its work. Fitness, exercise and body building have become big business for humans and human athletes and they have increased their physical output dramatically over the past decades. Humans choose to do this and often work with sports psychologists to create a 'winning' mental attitude. The horse wins because that particular horse is naturally bold and brave, quick and intelligent, capable and tough. Are we sometimes letting the horse down, isolating it and asking technical questions it can barely understand or cope with? The distance between the human desire to expand and the horse's own limits as an animal, which has no concept of great achievements but only of survival, can cause a great disturbance to the energy field in a horse on all levels. Sensitive horsemen and women will be aware of this. Many of the horses I see for healing have tried to express mental and physical discomfort and anyone who has studied the anatomy of the horse will marvel that we can ride them at all, as they are not physically very well structured. Owning and riding horses can bring great pleasure and satisfaction and I can honestly say the happiest moments of my life have been on horseback and the closest friendship I've had was with a horse. The more we tune in to the healing energies the more it will help us to understand the horse, its needs and our role in its life – helping us to answer some of the questions posed by this vocally silent friend and partner.

Environmental conditions

In our high-tech world we often forget that the horse is 'low tech'. No matter how much we advance in terms of science and how complicated our machines become, the horse remains a child of natural forces. Any interference we place in this path quite literally can screw up the horse's energy field – he has such a fine rapport with the universe and its messages. So many times I've come across horses who yearn to be kept like a horse and not like a car or a gadget. Things are, however, improving – as more and more people are realising what is important in their own journey through this life – and there is a growing interest now in healing as part of that enlightened approach.

The environment affects horses in a big way and can cause sometimes subtle, sometimes dramatic problems as these factors unsettle and unbalance the sensitive levels of energy within the horse. As with humans, some horses are more sensitive to, and therefore more affected by, environmental factors than others. The following environmental factors are particularly relevant to the horse:

❖ How they are kept.
❖ Where they are kept and their relationship to geopathic conditions.
❖ The weather and the seasons.
❖ Energy atmospheres and 'bad vibes'.

Geopathic conditions

Where horses are kept is an important factor and during my visits to give healing to horses I have noticed many things that can upset them. In their wild state, horses can move away from and avoid areas which they detect are creating energy havoc and blockages. They have no choice in captive conditions so it is something we need to be aware of. We cannot always move our horses because conditions are less than ideal but we can take steps to counteract the effects if these conditions affect any of them unduly.

Horses are very sensitive and capable of sensing geomagnetic fields, and these can affect biological rhythms, which healing may help to restore. The worst offenders in this category are electricity pylons. A few of my clients have pylons in their fields and have reported that some days they get static from the animals when they touch them and they also have to turn down the power of their electric fences. Plenty of research has been done into the potential effects these pylons can have on humans, including increase in tumours and depressed immune systems, and they can affect animals in a similar way. Healing is a natural therapy to consider to help counteract the negative influence of all that unusual electrical force in the air, and owners need to look out for increased health problems and depression in both themselves and their horses. Studies on humans in Germany and Austria have shown a correlation between serious illness, such as cancer, and geopathic stress zones. It is something to bear in mind when keeping horses and another reason to give horses healing, if conditions are less than ideal.

A couple of years ago I was asked to see a mare with severe heart disease. The mare's stable stood behind an electrical substation and a couple of pylons were also in the field so there was a lot of energy interference. I found the atmosphere very disturbing and within a couple of minutes had an unusual headache. The horse conveyed that she was very unsettled by the conditions in the field, which had made her feel more ill since being moved there the previous year, and the owner also confessed to feeling run down and depressed. Although the horse's heart condition was caused by malfunctioning valves the irritation from the pylons and substation was affecting the electrical energy in the heart muscle itself, making matters worse. The horse was moved and although still very ill was definitely brighter.

Stables built over ley lines, underground rivers and pipes, springs and mineral deposits can affect the horses kept in them. The work of healers and other therapists can be less effective over certain types of sub-surfaces, which can affect the reception of geophysical rhythms. The first time I came across this I was very puzzled. I was at a small-holding on a hillside surrounded by beautiful countryside and the horse was waiting for me in a large and comfortable stable. His owners had reported behavioural problems as well as continual recurring injuries. Usually I can go straight into 'healing mode' within seconds of stepping into the box and can detach my mind from any outside influences. This time, try as I might, I could not clear my head and concentrate. My thoughts were confused and I started to feel agitated. One of the horse's problems was that he was very fresh and irritable and I wondered if I was picking up on his feelings, so I stepped outside and my head quickly cleared. I asked for the horse to be moved to another stable block and was quickly able to function normally, giving a good healing treatment. The owners had built the stables themselves and knew that no previous buildings had stood there (past trauma in a building can affect the atmosphere). They were interested in dowsing so later on checked the stable and got a positive reading meaning a spring, stream or river was under it. This creates turbulence in the earth's magnetic field and was obviously affecting the horse. As a result that stable is now used as little as possible.

Energy atmospheres

Another very interesting incident has happened to me, which shows how past human behaviour can affect the atmosphere and create 'bad vibes'. I arrived at a remote farm and as I parked my car glanced at the house in front of the yard, which stood on raised ground, but noticed that it looked wrong somehow, and had a bad feel to it. As I stepped out of the car I suddenly couldn't breathe, and started to gasp horribly, feeling nauseous. I thought that I must be ill and stood by the car for several minutes until the feeling cleared, but I then felt so upset that I was tearful for a few minutes. I managed to pull myself together and walk to the small cottage in the grounds where I was to meet my clients.

The couple who met me were very nice and told me they were renting the facilities because the owner was away overseas. They had several horses for me to see; they were all much loved and well cared for, but I felt very sad inside myself as though I'd had some bad news. There were many empty outbuildings and I noticed that they were strange in design, some with huge doors, many with barred dark windows. The air hung thick with a horrible unnatural silence, and every now and then the wind blew, rattling a loose fixture as if to confirm the eerie feel of the place. I felt I needed to pray and did just that as I was giving the healing to the horses, as I felt a need to protect them from the atmosphere of this place. When I had finished I asked my clients who owned the property. They named a woman who had shortly before been prosecuted for distressing animal cruelty in a high-profile case, widely reported in the newspapers. It then all fell into place. I looked around at what I now realised were buildings that had housed bears, elephants, wild cats and chimpanzees and knew what was wrong. It was the past cries of imprisonment, fear, pain and distress whose energy hung heavy in the air that I could detect, and which made me feel so ill and depressed. I was very glad to leave that place.

The weather and the seasons

On every level of existence there is a complex network of various types of energy interaction. As well as existing in ourselves, and in animals, energies, rays or waves exist in plants, trees, insects and birds and have evolved since the beginning of the universe, constantly interacting with each other.

The horse has lost none of its sensitivity to subtle communications from the whole universe, including the tides, wind and weather, the sun, moon and the other planets. There are elemental energies of the earth itself relating to the seasons and the weather – measurable energies in water, air, fire and the ether (the aura of energies from all living things, which contain the blueprint of life). Weather-sensitive humans describe headaches, limb pain, sleep disorders, fatigue, confusion and indigestion, which can happen prior to changes in weather and which some sensitive horses can feel too.

In the 1950s, an eminent scientist and professor from Yale School of Medicine, Harold Saxton Burr, published a series of papers on how electric fields of animals and trees change in advance of changes in weather. Horses are very much affected by these conditions and by giving them an unnatural environment we can unbalance their equilibrium. This is another area where healing can play a role. Part of the complex nature of healing is to help restore balance to these horses – particularly where breakdown of response is caused by a restricted lifestyle.

The weather and the seasons can affect horses in many different ways and it is worth noting that research on humans has concluded that when a thunderstorm approaches there is statistically a greater chance of more frequent accidents, reaction times are slower and aggressive behaviour can increase. Horses can become frustrated when they do not have the freedom to act on the information that they receive through their instincts regarding changes in weather. They may, as a result, be punished for acting, for them 'naturally' but for the owners 'naughtily', and this becomes part of the complicated soup of disturbance that healers can pick up on when treating horses.

When a horse doesn't accept healing

When we offer healing to a horse it is important to let it know that our intent is to help and to ask permission from that horse to work with its spirit and body. It is not for us to dictate where that healing will go but to offer it to the horse where it is best needed, at whatever level. Rarely have I come across a horse that refused the healing, in fact, only twice in hundreds of cases. One was particularly sad and still haunts me.

A stud asked me to give healing to a brood mare as each time she was confirmed as being in foal she would reabsorb the foetus. This had happened on several occasions and vets could find no physical reason for her problem. The mare was valuable because in her earlier years she had won many competitions and races but a bad injury had put paid to her career. She had been scanned as being in foal again and the owner hoped that healing would help this time. The yard where I visited her was a good home but quickly into the healing treatment the mare told me of her early years when she had hated her life. During her youth of intensive stabling and stressful routine she had yearned for freedom, grass to roll on, wind to blow through her mane, sun to warm her back, friends to play with.

The mare turned to look me in the eye and I had that strong feeling of souls meeting. She told me she would never bring a foal into the world to live as she had done. I reasoned with her that there were good homes and kind owners, but she said she knew that it was a gamble where a foal would end up, it couldn't be guaranteed it would not be forced into the lifestyle she had so hated. She then sighed and thanked me for the tremendous peace that the healing had left her with. I passed this information on to the owner telling her that I knew the healing hadn't helped the mare physically but had given her spiritual and emotional peace. Sure enough, two weeks later a further scan showed that this foetus had been reabsorbed. Some months later the mare developed an incurable bone disorder and was put to sleep. It had a profound effect on me, teaching me that horses can and do make choices about their lives. They also play an active role in accepting healing on the level they know is best for them, which demonstrates just how complex their emotions are.

Healing as a preventative therapy

Earlier in the book I mentioned that healing is preventative and this has been shown in animal experiments, where the rate of wound repair was increased in animals given healing before injury. Each of the horse's systems is linked by a large number of interacting pathways and when in good health all these interactive and communicating channels produce co-ordinating actions. These include movement, respiration, wound repair, metabolism and digestion. Any malfunction of one pathway affects the whole, even though symptoms may not have appeared. Healing aims to restore the balance of the communicating and interconnecting channels, often working as a preventative measure.

People contact me regularly to visit a horse that does not have any apparent problems because they would like to know if the horse is happy and they want it to have healing for the therapeutic effects. A happy and balanced horse will be less prone to injury and disease and can recover more quickly in times of illness. But just because a horse is free of infection or disease does not mean that it is in good health. There can be many underlying health disturbances, some with a root cause a long time ago, some with a current cause. These disturbances can be on several levels and can result in problems in the future on any one or all of those levels. Illness and disease often have a root cause in the emotional level either from unbalanced thought or by the absorption of negative energy from others. What this means is that horses can become ill from stress and shock as well as bad handling. Their own thoughts can trigger a breakdown in homeostasis, or negative energy from handlers and riders can destabilise them. This is a good reason to have regular healing for your horse (and yourself too), as a preventative measure. That is not offering a guarantee that problems will not manifest themselves but with healing the horse should be better able to help itself overcome adverse conditions. The power of healing touch for the horse is very potent and very simple to access for anyone who wishes to help in this way.

For the competition horse, healing can enhance mental performance and concentration as well as helping to keep the body in better shape. This is because all the energy communication lines are open and in tune with each other. Healing also has a detoxifying effect – toxins can build up in the horse's body from either physical or emotional causes. These toxins can eventually depress the immune system or leave the horse feeling below par. Regular healing is beneficial as the deep relaxation and changes in energy flow which take place during a treatment can release these toxins. Human patients with a toxin build-up often report that they feel light-headed or headachy after healing and horses can probably feel the same way.

As a clairvoyant or intuitive healer I am able to pinpoint areas of energy weakness in the structure of the horse where problems could arise in the future. In these cases I will say to the owner, 'Keep a particular watch on that leg/foot/hock, etc.,' or even ask them to have investigations from the vet to check out what is going on. Often people report back, sometimes in as little as a week, sometimes in months, to tell me I was right and a problem had manifested itself. During healing, when I pick up these weaknesses, I will also be aiming to strengthen these areas so that if problems do manifest themselves the horse is better and more quickly able to recover.

Healing as a preventative measure

- ❖ Healing helps restore balance to all the systems.
- ❖ Emotionally blocked horses may suffer from more accidents and injuries in the future.
- ❖ Healing can help horses to express emotion.
- ❖ Healing can help the body to recover more quickly from illness and injury, and assists with soft tissue and bone repair.

4
Healing horses and the human link

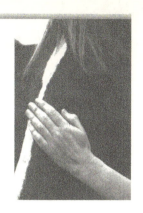

*'All things are bound together
All things connect
What happens to the earth
happens to the children of the earth
Man has not woven the thread of life
he is but one thread'*

        Anon

SOME PEOPLE ask me: is healing horses different to healing people? In my experience the answer to this question is yes and no, for several reasons. I can pick up through my hands similar responses when healing humans and horses but the energy field of the horse has different rhythms to the human energy field. Certainly the energy in the horse's cranio-sacral system and the relative pattern has a different cycle and rate to the human system. When I am giving healing to horses I often get much more sensation in my fingertips in terms of tingling, pulsing, hot and cold spots, etc. than I do when treating most humans and the reactions from the horses appear stronger and more evident. I also find it potentially more tiring, simply because of the focus and concentration involved to really get in tune with the horse's mental and emotional fields to facilitate the desired benefits. A human client is able to describe the problems physically, mentally and emotionally but the horse has no voice with human language to do this.

 Healing is offered to humans as much as it is offered to horses and it is up to the individual to accept the healing on some level, whether it is emotional or physical. At the end of the day it is up to the individual to accept the treatment or not, they have the final choice to let go. I find horses so very eager to take healing because they are so simplistic in their approach to life. Humans are much more complicated and can often have more

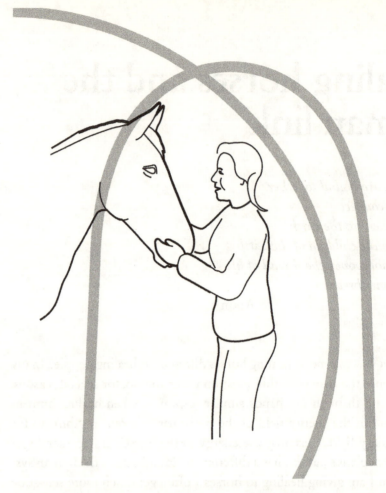

The shared energy of horse and human. Horses and humans have their own individual energy fields. As these radiate from the body so we also experience a 'shared energy', an overlapping or blending of one energy with another.

trouble clearing their minds or relaxing to enable them to absorb the re-balancing energy. Guilt, resentment, anger and hatred are all negative emotions, which can block the treatment. Sometimes, when an owner 'hangs on' to his or her emotional baggage it prevents the horse from being emotionally at peace. This is why I link both human and horse in a treatment, so that both benefit.

The energy that we have within us has our own individual pattern yet we all share a common energy, which overlaps and blends us subtly together. It appears that we can take on energy patterns and form from our horses too. A few years ago I went to an osteopath for cranial osteopathy to help whiplash problems sustained when I parted company with a horse at full gallop. During the treatment the osteopath, who also treated horses, said that I had a most unusual cranial rhythm, something he had not come across before. He went on to say it was part horse and part human and his comments made me take a good long look in the mirror afterwards. I don't look like a horse but my time spent giving healing to horses appears to mean that I have absorbed some of their energy patterns. The horses must be able to sense this as well because sometimes when I go up to a horse it looks startled as though it can't quite make me out – am I a human or a horse? The answer is that I am just a healer.

Another difference in healing horses is that they are black and white about responding to the treatment. They know what they feel in straightforward terms – hunger, pain, boredom, grief, anger, lack of company, frustration, the list is endless. I have found that when healing is offered the horse is usually willing to respond and the quickest area where healing is effective, and the easiest energy to release, is on an emotional level. This may be the hardest level to release for many people. I've found with the horse that when healing has facilitated an emotional release it usually stays cleared – provided, of course, that the environment and lifestyle is good for the horse. With people it appears that they may often hold on to their hang-ups, in some cases resurrecting them all again even as they climb off the treatment couch.

In my experience of giving healing to both horses and humans I have found that this unblocking of emotional energy can be quicker to effect in the horse and more often takes a few treatments in humans. There is an 'unwinding process', which for the horse operates on a simpler level than for humans. It is the complication of lateral and vertical thinking that results in a full release often taking longer for people. As a species we are more complicated, with more pressures and responsibilities, not least the fact that we are able to rationalise and analyse what is going on in our life – and there are, of course, many material, work, family and peer group distractions. The horse has simpler demands and appears to just want the feeling of being in balanced energy.

One big difference when giving healing to humans is that they are able to describe the sensations and reactions whereas with horses we have to rely on observational skills to know what is going on during a healing session. It is always extremely rewarding when a client tells of the benefits of healing treatment and how it has helped them move on in their life. It is through this information and feedback that I am able to build up a picture of how healing has helped the inner peace and sense of wellbeing of

Reactions to healing

Humans can cry and horses cannot, yet they feel the same emotion, and the horse seems so very grateful for the release of turbulent energy that healing offers it and is very willing to let go. I would go so far as to say that I have generally found that horses are more sensitive to energies and healing than many humans because they are more in tune with natural forces. Horses love healing and it is such an easy thing to offer for the benefit of the horse's inner peace, such a small part of our time, yet such a huge, dramatic and welcome experience for them.

Another difference when treating horses is that, of course, they are usually given healing while they are standing up and humans will be sitting or lying down. For this reason we need to be more careful and watchful with the horse. When the healing energy is very strong, the horse can become quite appear light-headed and unsteady on its feet and I've had to take my hands off many times to let a wobbly horse recover. I've never had to do this with a human, because if they become dizzy they are in a position whereby they are off their feet already anyway. I've observed that horses, like humans, can take several minutes to recover from this deeply relaxed state, and the changes can carry on taking place for quite a while after the actual healing session has finished. In some horses, after the release of deep-rooted trauma, this period can last several days. It is why I request that horses should be allowed to relax on the day that they have been given healing, just as a person would be advised to go home and take it easy.

horses. There is a 'wide circle' knock-on effect too, as the whole family will benefit when an individual is helped, just as a rider or owner will benefit when healing helps a horse and improvements are evident.

I always link humans and horses in the healing energy when I give a treatment as the shared energy must be rebalanced for the healing with the horse to be fully effective. It is the reason most clients will have strong energy responses when I am working with the horse. Not all healers work like this, but it is something that I have realised is very important, I would go so far as to say essential even, over the time that I have been specialising as an animal healer.

HEALING HORSES AND THE HUMAN LINK

To link the energy field of horse and human I always invite people to lay their hands on to the horse when I am giving healing. Frequently these people say that after a while it feels as though their hands are actually deep inside the horse. Sometimes people comment that there is a sensation as well of their hands 'being drawn into the horse' as if by a magnet. This is a fundamental human–horse healing link, of course, the attraction of electromagnetic energies one to the other. It is caused by the source of the blockage inside the horse (it may be the site of injury or disease) joining the bio-magnetic field of the healer. The human has offered the healing blue print – the missing link, which can establish homeostasis, balance of all the functions.

I think, perhaps, the major difference in healing horses as opposed to people is their innocence of verbal language and lack of any concept of self-image. People request healing for themselves because they are distressed, vulnerable and need help or, more fortunately, when there are no specific problems but just to keep them in good working order. The horse cannot directly request healing, but relies on someone being aware that the condition can be helped by hands-on healing. The horse is just as vulnerable as a human in need but it is not influenced by personalities, looks or ego. The horse responds simply to the healing rapport, whereas a human may respond as well to subtle messages from a strong personality and can be influenced by what the healer says, or their behaviour. Horses and other animals judge on what they feel and cannot be taken in by someone 'talking a good story, or putting on a show', so a positive reaction from them is evidence indeed that healing works. In short, there is absolutely no placebo effect in the response of horses to healing. If a person does not have good intent and ego is at the forefront of their personality it is of little use to the horse, which will instinctively resist and not absorb any healing. So we can see that to give healing to animals we need to be much more dedicated and deeply focused on them and their problems rather than on ourselves. They are great levellers in measuring our ability to do this.

Our own disturbed energy

Horses are very sensitive to and affected by our emotions, thoughts and intentions. These radiate as forms of energy from our minds and become part of the shared energy. Some horses are more sensitive than others and in adverse situations these horses can suffer undue stress, which in turn affects their own energy fields. I had first-hand experience of how much horses can 'read' our emotional energy a few years ago when out riding Goldie. We had been together for many years and I knew her inside out and presumably she me. It was high summer and I had arranged to ride in the evening after work, but during the afternoon had some terrible news. I felt in a state of shock but thought that a gentle ride in the country would be just the thing to help me relax and calm down.

As soon as I mounted Goldie she acted most strangely, flinging herself about and jumping from one side of the track to the other, becoming more and more erratic in her behaviour, exploding for no apparent reason. After a few hundred yards I dismounted for I understood then what Goldie was saying: 'Take that stressed, negative energy off my back and get yourself sorted because I don't like it.' I took her back to her paddock and then went home to arrange for some healing from a colleague. A couple of days later I felt much calmer and Goldie was perfectly happy to let me ride her again with no further objections to my energy state. Goldie was (she sadly died last year, aged 26 years) a dominant mare and therefore particularly sensitive to atmospheres and survival clues and she obviously had, quite rightly, decided that I was not in a fit state to look after myself or her. It was most interesting that the healing I'd had as a result of this incident rebalanced me enough to change her opinion on the next ride.

Another example of how our energy affects horses happened when I visited a yard to treat a young hunter – a valuable grey mare. I was told the horse had been owned for about a year but always became very agitated as soon as the rider got on and frequently threw her off. The mare would not let anyone touch her head and had become more and more aggressive when being handled from the ground. Before my visit I asked for the physiotherapist to check the back and saddle but nothing too bad was found.

As soon as I laid my hands on the horse she told me she was very depressed. She communicated that there was a very bitter and vindictive atmosphere around the owner due to a difficult divorce, which the horse hated, and the owner had also taken to drinking heavily, frequently riding with a hangover. The horse would not let her head be touched, she said, because it was her private space and she just wanted some peace in her life. Certainly I had no trouble laying my hands on the mare's head during the healing but when the owner stepped forward the horse pulled away. Bluntly I asked her about her personal problems in view of what the horse had told me but this lady unfortunately denied any stress in her life. However, the yard owner later confirmed that what I had picked up was true. After the healing, the little mare was very calm until a week later when her rider reappeared. Fortunately for the horse, the owner quickly lost patience and sold her, and after another healing session she settled very happily in her new home where she is not a problem to ride.

These stories are good examples of how we need to have healing ourselves to help horses cope when things are tough in our lives. Our thought energy has been scientifically shown to affect the mental health of people and animals in our care or our proximity. If you are having problems with your horse and your own life is troubled with negative emotions such as anger, depression, melancholy, resentment, impatience or grief, then try having a few sessions of healing yourself as well as arranging it for your horse. There should quickly be some improvements and benefits for both of you.

Children and healing

Children can be very sensitive to energy fields and I first became aware of my own healing abilities when I was a child. At the same time evidence of an intuitive/extra-sensory gift became apparent as well. I could 'see' things that others couldn't and I was aware of 'knowing' where there were areas of energy blockage in the bodies of both humans and animals, meaning that something was wrong. I was aware of feeling heat or tingling when I touched sick animals or people and could see colours as well, particularly a golden light around the whole body. As I grew older this was to refine itself until I could be more specific, for example to detect areas of pain and distinguish between emotional or physical blockage. Without knowing where or when I crossed another barrier and found that I could attune my mind to an animal's mind. A communication flowed and I found horses being the easiest to tune in to and through this communication I could pick up a cameo of their lives, giving a picture of emotional and physical health.

When I was a child, complementary medicine was practically unheard of and healing was considered on the fringe, whereas healing is now recognised within the National Health Service and by vets. Times certainly have changed – I never came across things like aromatherapy and reflexology until about 15 years ago and now most people are aware of these and other natural therapies, and healing has thankfully lost its eccentric image. I am very uplifted to find that many children and young people today are potential gifted healers too. Surprisingly regularly I come across such children in the places where I go to give healing to horses, the ages have ranged from two years upwards.

Subconscious abilities

William, a farmer's son, is a good example. I had gone to give healing to his mother's pony Sovereign to clear energy from a traumatic incident which had happened a couple of years previously. Some drunks had chased the pony down the road on its first trip out with a cart. I was just finishing when the boy appeared in the barn and watched me intently. With his mother's consent I invited him in to the stable and pointing to a place on the pony told him he could put his hand there. William, who was ten years old at the time and who did not know anything about me, touched the pony where I indicated and after a moment or two I said, 'Well, what do you think?' The boy pulled his hand away and smiling said, 'It's really weird, like electric shocks in my hand.' I asked him to touch another place and he had the same reaction.

To test him I asked him to place his hand over the sacral chakra and now he said, 'It's sort of the same but different – it's swirling round here like this,' and he described a circular movement on the horse. I was very impressed. The energy over the horse's sacral area is very active and has a lot of motion both circular and side to side. This rhythm has a very distinctive feel to it and in this particular pony it was very strong and this also has a swirling feeling under the hands. Finally I asked William to touch Sovereign's forehead, very gently. He stepped back after a couple of minutes and struggled to put what he felt into words. 'It was thinking, all his thoughts I could hear them. It was good,' he said finally. This was the area of the brow chakra and the centre of intuition and knowledge. Before I left, William placed both hands on the pony's back.

'It's working, healing is happening,' he said with all the innocence of a child. This was the first time the word healing had been mentioned and it came from him not me. I went on to treat the family dog and William described seeing a golden light under my hands as I treated, evidence that he was seeing the dog's aura. With his mother's supervision William now often gives healing to Sovereign and other animals on the farm, which is a wonderful thing and bodes well for the future of mankind.

Several other children have described seeing light under my hands, some pointing out different colours as I move them around the horse. Always they have accurately described chakra colours or colours which have corresponded to blockages in the aura relating to various conditions. Other children have picked up feelings or thoughts from the ponies as the healing has taken effect. None of these children had a clue what they were describing and frequently had not heard about healing. In some cases the parents were in fact initially sceptical of my work and had called me as a last resort.

It is good that today there is now so much interest in natural remedies and treatments and a desire to get back to our spiritual roots, the foundation of which is, of course, healing, the oldest and purest form of medicine. These young people, already showing strong healing abilities have, I believe, a special future role to play with the welfare of humans, horses and other animals.

Jemima's healing powers

Another potential healer is Jemima, who comes from a particularly environmentally caring family. When I met her she was also ten years old. Her mother asked me to see the girl's beautiful new pony, Cally, to help it settle with them as it had come to them from a long way away. As I laid my hands on the pony I felt waves of sadness and at the same time Jemima let out a heartrending sound, 'Oh, Mummy – she's so sad. I can feel how upset she is and there are so many tears,' and Jemima wept softly. The pony was tense to start with but now became very still. After a few minutes a feeling of intense calmness descended all around us and the pony and Jemima sighed together. There would now always be a special bond between them as Cally knew that the girl had shed her tears for her, so that she could be at peace. Jemima described how she had picked up the pony's emotions during the healing as though she was the pony. She is a girl who goes around placing her hands on people and animals 'to make them better', a sure sign of a gifted healer in the making.

Horses who lead me to people who need healing

There have been many times when I've gone to give healing to a horse and a person associated with that horse has needed healing as well. Through treating the horse and linking the human both have been helped. These are the times when the horse has led me to people who need healing, situations where that person would not otherwise have considered or thought that healing could help their particular problem. The response of the horse has stimulated the person involved to want to participate in the healing for a benefit to themselves.

One such situation occurred when I went to see a beautiful chestnut gelding called Oro (which means gold in Spanish). It was the second time that I'd visited the horse, which the vet had diagnosed as suffering from a severe allergic reaction, and I was giving healing treatments to help raise the immune system. On this second visit, just as I was just about to start, a man in a wheelchair suddenly buzzed into the yard. My client introduced him as Phil, her husband, and I felt that there was more work to be done that day than treat the horse. Phil sat watching me and said that he was fascinated by what I had come to do – his wife had explained the reactions of the horse during my last visit and her own responses as she held the rope. 'Come over, Phil, and take a contact,' I said, 'if you would like to share in the healing.'

Phil, who I guessed to be in his forties, moved his chair closer to the stable door and I placed the rope in his hands as his wife stood to one side of him. I placed my hands on Oro's back – he was a model patient – and tuned in to the healing energy. Now Oro is a particularly sensitive horse with a highly active energy field. I had noted during my first visit that I had to take my hands off several times as he became so wobbly on his legs. So I made sure that I directed the energy flow through gently and after a couple of minutes I glanced across at Phil. I looked down at the rope and could see golden light shooting along the rope like it was on fire.

The aura of energy I saw was powerful and strong and I looked back at the horse – he was showing signs of endorphin response, his head drooping and his eyes closing. 'I feel light-headed,' Phil suddenly said. 'That's a good response,' I replied, not expecting what happened next. Phil promptly dropped the rope and fainted, slumping forward in his chair. His wife is a highly qualified nurse and she moved to help him so I wasn't alarmed, but I knew something very special had responded to Phil's desire to experience

HEALING HORSES AND THE HUMAN LINK

the healing. After a few minutes Phil was bright again and said, 'I want more, please, can I have the rope back.' So I carried on and at the end of the session Phil said that his neck pain had gone and that he felt energised.

I was very pleased to be able to help this man, who has spent more than twenty years in a wheelchair after a motor racing accident. The healing energy, which had channelled from me through the horse and out to the man, had taken on an added power and the beneficial effects to Phil lasted for several days.

Then there was Tina, who didn't tell me when I went to give healing to her horse that she had a history of depression. One of the reasons that she called me to treat her mare was that the horse was in low spirits due to bad treatment in a previous home. I guess Tina felt a subconscious sympathy with the mare's depression, having spent years with a black cloud of her own which never seemed very far away. Tina was certainly very intuitive and in touch with her horse's feelings and mind. The horse responded very well to the healing treatment and there were lots of positive releases and signs that she would feel much improved. As always, I asked her owner to place her hand on the mare as I worked so that she could see what she picked up of the healing energy and Tina reported a lot of reactions.

A week later Tina rang me. Her horse had never appeared better. For a day after the healing the mare was quite exuberant, as though she couldn't believe how different she felt, then she settled into a calmness, which had remained. But Tina also wanted to tell me of something strange that had happened to her after my visit. The next morning she had woken with her cloud of depression there as bad as it had ever been. For two days she felt bad, but something was different this time, she felt that she could cope. On the third day the depression had suddenly gone and she felt fantastic. I explained that the healing she shared with her horse must have worked to clear out her own emotional blockages releasing that disturbed energy and clearing it away. A year later Tina and her horse still feel very happy and are enjoying a new lease of life together.

These are just two examples of horses that have led me to people who need healing but there have been many more such cases. Our lives are interwoven and linked with our horses with which we share an energy in this world. I believe that there is a great deal to discover and to learn about the purpose of our shared journey. With improved empathy there is much more help that we can give our horses and in return receive from them. We only need to open our hearts and minds.

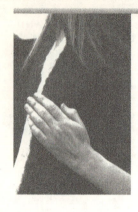

5
Case histories

*'Gentle, vegetarian,
intelligent and brave,
the horse for countless centuries
has been man's friend and slave'*
    from *The Horse* by Vernon Scannell

The following is a selection of case histories and I have included ones that give a good cross section of the conditions and problems experienced by most horse owners and riders. The case histories have been grouped under subject headings for ease of reading and identification, although more than one topic may be covered. Some of the stories are sad and some are uplifting. I hope that all of them will give an added insight to the horse and demonstrate that healing is a journey into the spirit of the horse. In some instances names have been changed at the request of clients.

OVERCOMING BEHAVIOURAL PROBLEMS

Fanta's barrier

This case history could also have appeared in the section of the elderly horse (see page 96) as Fanta was 24 years old when I gave her healing and demonstrates how long horses can be emotionally damaged by ill treatment. For the last ten years of her life, Fanta had lived with several other ponies, horses, dogs and cats with a very caring lady called Val. As I stepped close to Fanta, a very pretty chestnut Anglo-Arab, I immediately picked up pain around the ears and a feeling of being twitched there at some time in the past. She communicated that she'd known periods of real hunger and there was depression in there as well – after nearly 20 years she still felt a deep sense of loss over a foal. Fanta communicated that she'd had two foals and it was the second one she longed for and missed. It had died at around four months old in unpleasant circumstances and the mare had always wondered where it went.

Although the horse appeared quite friendly I knew that there was a barrier around her which I hoped the healing treatment would remove. Val knew nothing of Fanta's previous history but said she would try to find out. Val did tell me that in the ten years she'd had the horse, neither she nor anyone else had been able to touch Fanta's ears. She had tried everything but the horse would fling her head up and run backwards as soon as someone reached up to touch the head and ears. I gently laid a hand on Fanta's neck and she turned to me looking deeply into my eyes. A heavy presence descended around us, and in those very humble stable surroundings I suddenly felt the power of God's love stand and watch over us. Fanta coughed and snorted, then she began to show the usual endorphin reaction of becoming very sedated, swaying softly and slowly as I kept a contact with my fingertips. The horse turned to me again and our eyes fused in question and answer, in space and time – in love from the giver to the receiver. She turned away and looked ahead for a moment before sighing and letting her head drop to the floor. She had let go.

At this point Val said she felt light-headed and very sad so she stepped away for a moment or two to get her equilibrium back. I then asked Val to touch my hand where I had it placed on Fanta's neck and asked her what she could feel. Straight away she said that she could feel tingling up her arm, then it travelled to her feet. I explained that was the healing energy and that Fanta would feel it too. There were three other people watching and all were sceptical at first but they experienced similar sensations. Fanta became very peaceful at the end of the session and allowed me to place a hand on her forehead to channel healing through the brow chakra, but I stayed away from her ears.

The next evening Val rang to say she was ecstatic, there had been a major improvement in Fanta overnight. Val had gone into her stable the next morning and something made her touch the horse's ears. Fanta dropped her head in approval and with her heart in her mouth Val softly rubbed the ears. The horse remained calm and closed her eyes in happiness. Val was so excited she spent 20 minutes touching and grooming Fanta's head and ears and still Fanta stood still and didn't push her away. Since the healing Fanta now loves a cuddle and to have her ears stroked. 'Fanta is softer and

> **The horse turned to me again and our eyes fused in question and answer, in space and time – in love from the giver to the receiver.**

happier. She looks forward to me grooming her now and calls to me. Healing definitely took the barriers away and her bad memories,' said Val.

Eighteen months later I heard from Val again. She had been able to trace Fanta's previous owners who said that the mare had always been head shy so they had frequently twitched her ears for dental work, mane trimming, head grooming, etc. This was evidence of the communication from the horse about pain and shock that she had suffered in the past. The changes from the healing have been permanent and Fanta is still happy now to have anyone touch her head and ears.

Bejay's self-mutilation

Bejay was a six-year-old who his present owner had bought from an overseas dealer about six months before she contacted me. The horse had passed through at least six previous homes and he was very uptight. He loved his work though and had won several championships with his new owner, an expert and well-known horsewoman. This lady said to me that the least she could do to reward Bejay was to help him find peace and she felt something awful must have happened to him in the past. He would trash his stable when in he was in it, and twice it had been completely rebuilt. Thick padding covered the walls from floor to ceiling to help prevent the little horse from injuring himself.

When Bejay was let out into the paddock with the other horses he would gallop off and then stop dead. He then would proceed to tear strips of flesh from anywhere he could reach on his body, self-mutilating to show his disgust at whatever dark secrets the past held. The vet had no solution for such a troubled animal. Bejay stood in his stable when I first visited as tense and rigid as though he was made of plastic and he flinched when I moved. The horse communicated what had happened to him when he was broken as a three-year-old, how he was left tied up in his stable for months and deprived of food and water to break his spirit. Water was offered daily by the handler and when he was dehydrated he would take some, thereby being taught that man was in control of his whole life and needs. He had hated all stables ever since because of this and hated his body because of the control mankind had over him. The horse would never drink in his stable and would only drink from buckets in the field. Because of his destructive nature he had been sold on from person to person, each one unable to stop him. Bejay knew that the new owner was aware of his emotional needs and loved him, but he didn't know how to let go of his anger.

I put my fingertips on the horse's neck to start the healing properly but he raised his head in fear, becoming more rigid. Speaking softly to Bejay I channelled the healing deep into his solar plexus area to begin with and as I did so he stood rooted to the spot with his head slightly bent watching me as I worked my fingers over his body. I knew the horse would be worried by the strange sensations he felt from the healing energy but I was pleased when he began to show signs of accepting the feeling of sedation, his eyes flickering. For a while the horse became more agitated and started pulling at his owner's jacket with his lips while she reported a feeling of being light-headed and a tightness in her chest. I knew that horse and rider were linking together in an exchange of energy, then it hit me too with a thud as a wave of tears came out of the horse. Years of frustration, pain and anger came away as the negative energy which humans express as tears discharged. The horse's owner felt it too and she became emotional at this point.

As I gently touched Bejay's left hip he started to sway, a slow gentle rhythm until the movements got bigger and bigger and he staggered. I moved my fingertips to the horse's forehead and he leaned on the wall to support himself. Twenty minutes after I began he was calm and peaceful. He looked smaller, his body soft and round where it had been hard and tense. The skin, especially around the neck, was dramatically softer and looser. Bejay's owner looked bemused as she watched her horse. 'There is already a difference,' she said as she watched him in what I call 'healing time'. As I drove away, she stood in amazement as he calmly went to his water bucket and, for the first time in six months, drank slowly and deeply, savouring every drop.

Bejay looked very different during my second visit and had not self-mutilated or trashed his stable since his healing session. The second time I saw him he was like a pussycat in the stable and he was so relaxed and sociable I hardly recognised him. He was calling to his owner and licking our hands. The horse was much more relaxed to treat on this occasion and his owner experienced tingling sensations in her hands as she held him. Everyone who knows the horse says, 'Bejay has his peace now,' which is exactly what his owner had wished for and he has never displayed any behavioural problems again.

> I knew that horse and rider were linking together in an exchange of energy, then it hit me too with a thud as a wave of tears came out of the horse.

Mincala's depression

This very interesting horse was given healing by me in less than ideal circumstances. I had been invited to do a lecture demonstration for a riding club, which used the facilities of a large college. More than 80 people had assembled to watch me talk and demonstrate healing including several professionals in the equestrian field and a senior local vet. I had asked the organiser to arrange for three horses to be used for the evening. In the end he brought three with behavioural problems, none of which showed any physical reason for their unhappiness when examined by their vets. As I arrived in the large indoor school where the event was being held, I saw the horses waiting patiently with their owners along one side of the hall. At the other side sat the audience. The whole environment was less than ideal for my healing, bright fluorescent lights, lots of distractions not to mention having to talk during most of the healing demonstrations to explain what was happening. But nevertheless I was there to do a job and rise above these things.

Just before I started, as the organiser was introducing me, I turned to look at the horses – I felt emotional, they all needed healing and looked me in the eyes to ask for help. I got up to give my talk and suddenly thundering rain started to beat down on the plastic roof, deafening everyone. They could not hear me so there was a chaotic few minutes as the audience moved their seats further forward, and still the horses stood behind me watching me.

Rebecca brought the first horse, Mincala, an eight-year-old bay thoroughbred mare, forward to me. As the horse stood next to me I felt her emotional pain and distress; she was very stressed by something that had happened in the past. Rebecca had owned Mincala for 18 months and she confirmed that she was very tense, box walking all night so that in the morning her stable had to be completely cleared out as it was in such a mess. Rebecca described her as a lunatic in the show jumping ring, running around with her head in the air, and the slightest thing would upset her terribly. All Rebecca's patience and kindness had not helped this mare to let go of the stress from her past. Under the circumstances, with everyone watching, I found it difficult to tune in to Mincala's thoughts properly to find out what exactly had happened. I knew enough to start the healing, though – I was dealing with shock, tension and depression.

All the time that Mincala had been standing by me she looked tense, her body was stiff and she had a wary look in her eye. I stepped forward to lay my hand on her neck and she stepped away, so I spoke to her gently and asked her to let me help release the pain. Within a few seconds she softened and showed the tell-tale signs of endorphin release as the healing started its powerful effects. I wanted to be quiet and absorb what was happening but I had to carrying on talking and explaining to the people watching me. It was like trying to listen to several conversations at once.

Twenty minutes later, Mincala stood absolutely still with her head hanging down as she swayed and sighed in peace. I said, 'Well, we have a big energy change in this horse.' Suddenly someone in the audience called out, 'And look at the rider, look at the change in her too.' I turned to look and saw that Rebecca was pale and appeared as sleepy as her horse. They slowly left the arena and I went on to complete the evening. At the end, Rebecca's parents came up to me and said that as their daughter had got to the horse lorry with Mincala she felt a sharp pain in her neck and was suddenly light-headed too. They added that the year before she'd had a serious accident and had damaged her neck with subsequent recurring problems. I explained that Rebecca had shared the healing too and the reactions she had felt were the changes in the energy field as everything rebalanced.

Three months later I heard from the family again – they were absolutely delighted and wanted to know when I was in that area again. They had noticed a personality change in Mincala the day after I'd given her healing. From being unrideable, Mincala had just come third in the riding club special beginners points listing – all accumulated since the healing treatment that evening. The changes in the horse's temperament also meant that Rebecca was able to hack the horse out on her own. Mincala was very good to ride in the show jumping ring now and didn't get upset any more or panic if things went wrong, staying calm and jumping many clear rounds. Rebecca said, 'She's very laid back now and happier in herself, with an inner peace I've not seen before. We had a catastrophic year last year and I'm thrilled to be able to do so much with her now. Also I haven't had any pain in my back, which is a bonus too.' Her mum had the last word. 'If the healing worked like that in a demonstration, what would it be like on a one to one?'

I stepped forward to lay my hand on her neck and she stepped away, so I spoke to her gently and asked her to let me help release the pain.

Conker's mood changes

The first time I saw Conker I fell in love, for he is a very handsome big black five-year-old sport horse. Although a young horse, the look in his eye acknowledged pain and disappointment that were beyond his years. Annie had owned him for a couple of months when she called in equine physiotherapist Jo Verhaeg to assess his physical condition. Conker had been well bred in Ireland and shipped over to England as a yearling, ending up with a lady who wanted him for hunting. Consequently as a three-year-old he was quickly broken and did 40 days' hunting before he was four. Something went horribly wrong and the horse was put up for sale, 'surplus to requirements'. That's where Annie came on to the scene and, hearing about the young black horse, went to see him. It was love at first sight for her too. She asked if the horse had had any falls or injuries and told none at all. The horse was fat and had no muscle tone as well as having a dreadful coat – harsh and dull.

Conker alternated between depressed and agitated so Annie brought him on slowly, hacking him out quietly around the country lanes. She eventually hoped the horse would do well in show jumping, which was her main interest. When Conker was ridden he would suddenly and for no apparent reason get moody and become very irritable, charging off dangerously for ten minutes or so before settling into a frantic jog. He did a couple of unaffiliated competitions and showed real promise, getting into the jump-offs. But all was clearly not well and he became very stiff on the left rein and very blocked in the neck as well as weak behind. More worrying was that the behavioural problems were getting worse and he was displaying frequent bouts of anger. When Jo Verhaeg first assessed him she considered that his musculo-skeletal problems were so bad that he would need manipulation under general anaesthetic. However, he was happy to be treated by Jo and responded well to her mobilisation techniques. After a couple of sessions Jo felt that she was making good progress physically but that the horse had huge emotional problems creating tension, which was holding back full physical recovery.

Conker had been with Annie for ten months when I first saw him and he conveyed several things to me. Firstly that he was missing a special friend that he had made in his previous home, and secondly that he'd had a terrible accident out hunting, when he had fallen on his head. He was suffering bad headaches and his mood swings happened when a black cloud seemed to suddenly descend over him making him feel angry. Annie said that was a good description of his moods. He also communicated that ill treatment and his fighting back to it resulted in being hit about the head and being tied tightly down to a martingale. He is a horse who likes to push people to the limit – cheeky joker – and being previously with an insensitive person had been punished for it. I also picked up that he is insecure and indecisive so needed a confident rider, which he now fortunately had. As a result of all this confusion his behaviour had become more and more erratic.

I started the healing treatment as I usually do by softly laying my hand on his neck. Within a couple of seconds Conker closed his eyes. Everything was very peaceful as I gradually moved my hand to the chest where I would work through the solar plexus. Annie suddenly said she wanted to cry as a rush of emotional energy left the horse and Conker was able to let go of things he had bottled up for so long. He started to sway and he was obviously feeling peaceful and after ten minutes or so his skin was looser and softer. I walked round to his side and laid my hands on the middle of his back. After a minute or so there was a wave of movement along his spine as a kinetic release of energy took place and Conker's back dropped. When I put my hands gently on his head he turned towards me and sighed, his eyes tightly closed. He became absolutely still and at this point my fingertips became very tingly with a terrific heat building up under my hands, which Annie could feel as well. At the end of the treatment Conker yawned deeply and when I left the look in his eye was much more peaceful.

I saw Conker again a couple of weeks later and the outlook was very positive. The day after his healing Annie had noticed huge beneficial changes. He was altogether a much sweeter person and was making friends with the other horses as well. Jo treated him with physiotherapy a couple of times more and found that the emotional release from the healing had helped his physical progress enormously – he did not need to be treated under general anaesthetic and she was quickly able to sign him off as absolutely A1. Annie was able to research the horse's background and confirm the accident that I picked up from him. Someone she met had seen his fall, exactly as I had described it. Conker is now a confident, cheeky, fit and happy horse without any mood swings and he is doing fantastically well in his work, enjoying his jumping career.

At the end of the treatment Conker yawned deeply and when I left the look in his eye was much more peaceful.

William's unpredictability

William came to one of our Top to Toe days and the change in him after healing was dramatic and instant. He had competed in dressage with his owner Katie and reached the National Championship at elementary level a couple of years before. He was brought for treatment as Katie found him a problem horse, being mentally very difficult. He was either very angelic or very bad tempered, and Katie found she had to be several steps ahead of him as he was very strong and stubborn. Most riders would have found the horse terrifying as he was so unpredictable, but Katie loved him and wanted desperately to know what was bothering him and to help him find some peace. When I stepped into the box with William he was very apprehensive, and swishing his tail he barged around crossly. Katie had a job to hang on to the rope as he dragged her around the stable but eventually he stopped and stood watching me anxiously. I quickly picked up that he often had a great deal of pain in his right jaw and the poll energy was twisted. He had nervous spasms in his intestines and the stomach area had a blockage of energy.

The horse was also a manic worrier, was antisocial and withdrew into himself focusing on his problems, therefore becoming more and more depressed. To top it all he lacked confidence – altogether a complicated character and a challenge to help. Katie confirmed that as a youngster the horse had a nasty accident which hurt his back and head (he was having physiotherapy) and which could account for the face pain.

I had to be slow and patient when giving healing to William, as any sudden movements made him worry, but after a while he became much less tense. My aim with him was for the healing to give him some emotional release, which would help him let go of negative energy, and by relaxing him to release some physical tension. The horse began to lick and chew in acceptance and his outline softened considerably as he allowed some moments of sedation, closing his eyes and sighing. When they went home that day Katie noticed that he was much calmer and appeared less stressed. Normally he was a worried traveller but he was more relaxed about that too.

Two days after the healing Katie took William to a dressage lesson and he was the best he'd ever been. Normally she had to fight him all the time but suddenly she didn't have to. Her instructor, a top dressage rider who'd taught them both for a long time, couldn't believe the difference. I saw the

> **My aim with William was for the healing to give him some emotional release, which would help him let go of negative energy, and by relaxing him to release some physical tension.**

horse again two weeks later and he was much calmer and easier to work with. He was very responsive to the healing and sleepy at the end of the session. A month later William and Katie were chosen for the British Pony Club dressage team to compete at the European Championships in Ireland. 'William was very relaxed and was a dream to ride,' said Katie, 'and we were thrilled that our team won, something previously I would never have believed possible.'

Ratty's feeding problems

YOUNG EQUINES

It is never too early to give healing to a horse and none are too young. I have been giving healing to Ratty and her foal from when the mare was three months pregnant. Ratty is a chestnut thoroughbred mare and had a lot of problems when she gave birth last time. She has particularly sensitive skin and cannot bear anyone to touch her underneath her belly. Her owners had stayed up for hours when they knew the birth was imminent and were alarmed to see that as soon as the foal, a filly, got up to suckle, Ratty moved away and wouldn't let it suckle. The vet was called who sedated Ratty and she was milked so that the first vital drink containing colostrum could be bottle-fed to the foal. For a few hours try as they might the owners could not settle Ratty to let her foal take more milk, she just moved away around the stable. It was a terribly stressful morning but gradually Ratty felt happier about feeding the foal and things quickly got better to the point where she allowed her to suckle.

Some time later I was visiting Ratty's home to treat another horse for post-viral syndrome and we thought it would be useful to start giving Ratty some healing while she was in foal. As I laid my hands on her she quickly responded and became very calm and sleepy. Suddenly I could feel the foal in her womb link in to the healing and start to jiggle. Then a tremendous feeling of warmth filled my hands and I felt as though I was holding the foal in them, which now was very still. It was a most magical moment to feel the response of this developing life to the healing. I treated Ratty again a month later and this time I could 'see' the foal lying in the womb as I placed my hands on the mare's side. The foal was large and strong and as I started the healing it jiggled again with pleasure.

Then a tremendous feeling of warmth filled my hands and I felt as though I was holding the foal in them, which now was very still.

I mentioned what I had picked up about the foal and Ratty's owner confirmed that it made sense, for she then told me that the stallion was a big-boned Swedish dressage horse. At the time of writing I continue to see Ratty – her foal will be born the month that this book is published and I am very much looking forward to the birth.

Mr Bumble's laboured breathing

At just ten days old, Mr Bumble is one of the youngest equines I have given healing to. I was visiting a place to treat a pony and horse when the very proud owners asked me if I would have a look at their donkey foal. Within the last 24 hours he'd started to breathe heavily and pant. Obviously the vet had checked him, but when I went in to see the little chap I felt that he had a headache. He was lying down looking distressed and I asked the owners if he'd had anything around his neck or head. I was concerned to hear that since two days of age a head collar had been used (a halter called a foaling slip) to lead him into the stable at night and out again in the morning. This is potentially dangerous for such a young foal as the individual skull bones are very soft and can easily get compressed or distorted. Also a tug on the rope can damage the poll and cervical bones and even dislocate the neck. I explained to the owners a safer way to move a foal around, and then asked permission from the foal's mother Joan to treat her baby, whereupon she obligingly stepped aside.

I had to be quick with my treatment so as not to distress the foal and I placed the thumb and forefinger of each hand around the front and back of the ears to target the healing into the head. Within a couple of seconds his eyes flickered shut and his little legs wobbled. I took my hands away and waited a minute or two for the foal to settle before doing the same thing again. The donkey's eyes again closed tightly and after about another minute I stopped the treatment – healing is very powerful in something so young. The foal rocked backwards and forwards then began to lick and chew, his tiny lips making a soft sound. Mr Bumble's breathing had become much more normal and he turned to look up at me, his huge ears flicking forward quizzically. Then with a swish of the tail he went to drink from his mother. I checked on Mr Bumble a week later and he was very well and much happier. So much so that at four months he went on to win best foal in a show, and together with his mother took the cup for best mare and foal.

Like many youngsters, Mr Bumble sometimes injures himself or takes a tumble in the field. His owner John was very keen to explore his hands-on healing abilities so that he could use healing as soon as something happened. During the course of a few visits I instructed John in how to give healing to Mr Bumble, showing him where to place his hands and talking him through the various sensations and responses. John has since practised healing very successfully and, having several horses, ponies and donkeys, has used it on all of them for various reasons. John has had some excellent results and is a very good example of an owner discovering and developing their own healing potential. 'I find it very rewarding and give healing every day if there is a problem. I feel as though I am doing something positive and I can certainly feel the sensations of the healing energy flow through my hands.'

When I am called to do some healing work on his animals John will now join me by placing his hands on the patient at the same time. This boosts the healing energy, and is also a happy sharing of the experience.

Rufus's epilepsy

Sometimes I have been at a place treating a horse when another one has become ill and I have given healing as first aid. Rufus was such a case. I was just completing a treatment to a mare when there was a terrific squealing and whinnying from the field behind the stable I was in. Rufus, a grey horse, was in a full epileptic seizure and was collapsing on to his knees. The screaming and whinnying was coming from his companion, a small black and white pony called Liquorice. Liquorice had his head underneath Rufus's neck as he was falling down and was desperately trying to support him and keep him from falling. Rufus was shaking from head to toe and his eyes were rolling back into his head. He dragged himself up, then his back legs buckled and he started to fall sideways – Liquorice pressed his body against the grey horse and staggering himself helped him as much as he could. Over and over again Rufus staggered and fell and his friend stayed with him to help. Sometimes both horse and pony fell down and would scramble to their feet, Rufus's body in spasms. The centre of the field had some jumps in, and a pile of poles. Rufus stumbled over them and we started to drag them clear. The groom said she would call the vet and went back to the house.

Very carefully I walked close to the stricken horse. He was pleading for help. His body was in convulsions, his neck twisted, his tongue hanging down. His eyes met mine and I have never seen such fear. Keeping a watch for my safety I reached out and placed a hand on the horse's neck. For several minutes we stuck together – as he twisted and fell and thrashed around I moved with him, keeping a contact with my hand. Many times he fell to the ground but I kept the healing going and I could feel the very disturbed energy pulsing through my fingers. After about ten minutes Rufus became calmer and eventually became more steady on his feet so I moved my hand to his head and for a minute or two I stayed in this position, the horse's eyes fixed on mine. Then the moment of seizure had passed, the horse was obviously distressed and shaky, but otherwise OK. I stepped back and slowly he started to walk round and round the field, Liquorice following close on his heels. The vet checked Rufus over and could find no damage to the horse but he was retired from being ridden.

> I could feel the healing beginning to take effect and the horse's breathing rate began to slow right down.

Just under two years later I was asked to treat Rufus again. Since my last visit he'd been well but was starting to have fits again. When I put my hands on the horse, as I expected, the energy field felt like a swarm of bees. Amazingly, within a second or two of placing my hands in position Rufus let out a long sigh and a short time later his back suddenly dropped a couple of inches. I could feel the healing beginning to take effect and his breathing rate began to slow right down. At this point his owner suddenly said she was very light-headed and a pulse went throughout her body. I could feel a definite change in cranial energy rhythm at the end of the treatment. Regular healing certainly helps the horse's epilepsy and his owners report that Rufus is always very much happier and brighter for a few weeks after a treatment.

Zara's weight loss

When Zara, a 16-year-old thoroughbred mare, experienced a sudden and dramatic weight loss her owner Kay called me to see if I could help. She was a horse I had seen several months before when I had very successfully given a couple of healing treatments for behavioural problems. Zara is an ex-racehorse and had always been nervy and flighty. She had been difficult to catch and had never liked being tied up. After I had given the horse just one healing session for her behavioural problems Kay was thrilled to report an immediate and dramatic improvement. As I started the

CASE HISTORIES

first healing treatment Kay was worried that Zara would lash out. As I touched her as she was very ticklish but with me she relaxed and gradually fell asleep as the healing took effect. Zara then let go of a lot of unhappiness from the past, which enabled her to have a much more positive outlook on life from then onwards. Overnight she also became affectionate and more trusting, which allowed Kay to do more things with her.

So Kay decided to call me in again when Zara became sick. Her weight had gradually dropped over several weeks and the vet had run lots of tests, which didn't show anything. Nothing could be found to cause the sudden thinness and lack of vitality. Zara became thinner and Kay discussed treatment from me with her vet who is very open-minded to complementary therapies. And thin Zara certainly was – when I saw her again she looked pitiful with bones sticking out everywhere and her head like a skull. Kay had spent a small fortune on expensive food and supplements to build up the horse and try to get the weight back on, but Zara appeared very lethargic as she stood in front of me. It was a bitterly cold winter's day and Zara had several layers of duvets and rugs covering her to keep her warm.

I touched the sides of the horse's body over the rugs, gradually working my way around her body. After a while I picked up an energy blockage in the immune system and some minutes later I felt the energy start to move, slowly at first then more quickly like a stream starting to flow. Suddenly there was a kinetic release – and her tail jerked up, then she was peaceful again. I saw Zara once more two weeks later and she was looking much better. Kay reported that the horse was more like her old self and within a couple more weeks the weight had stabilised and Zara went on to make a full recovery.

Suddenly there was a kinetic release – and her tail jerked up, then she was peaceful again.

Theo's sudden head-collar fear

I was asked to go and see if I could help Theo, a little New Forest pony, by a vet. When I first met Theo he was just 12 months old, a very nice example of his breed and a pretty roan colour. He had been bred wild in the New Forest National Park and spent the first four months running free with his mother, then he was brought in for one of the autumn pony sales. Jackie had bought him from the auction when he was five months old. She had gone to look for a youngster, having recently lost her very elderly

TRAUMATISED AND SHOCKED HORSES

89

riding pony. Although he had been weaned too early and quickly Theo settled in really well and for three weeks he was happy and calm.

One night as she was sitting in her kitchen at around midnight Jackie had a sixth sense that something was very wrong with Theo. Then suddenly the dogs started barking furiously and taking a torch Jackie went out and crossed the yard to the paddock. She heard a tremendous commotion and in the torchlight saw Theo thundering from one side of the field to the other. His head was up, his eyes were rolling and he was galloping wildly, stumbling and falling as he went. Jackie called to him and eventually he slowed up. As she went nearer to the pony she could see the horror and terror in his eyes. Every time she went towards her normally placid pony he ran off in fear, and when she lifted her hand to put on the head collar he flinched – something he had never done before. He was shaking from head to foot and covered in sweat. What had happened to him?

For the next couple of weeks Jackie couldn't go near Theo and eventually she called in his original breeder to get the head collar back on. He chased the pony round eventually cornering him and grappling with him to get it round his head. Jackie led Theo to his stable and was very upset – a dramatic and sudden character change had taken place and he was extremely nervous. If a man approached he ran wildly away, having previously been calm with men. A couple of weeks later Theo got the head collar off again in the paddock and he would not let Jackie near him to put it on. Not wanting to upset him she left him, hoping he would calm down. She got him a friend, a little grey pony, and Theo loved him to bits, so he would follow this pony into the stables and paddocks and by this method Jackie could move him around. Time went on, however, and Theo didn't become any more peaceful – something terrible had happened to him and he was in shock.

When I saw Theo he had been like this for eight months. He was in the stable when I arrived, having followed his friend into it. He was very nervous and I stood outside for a while talking to his owner. She opened the door and stepped in but when I tried to follow he rushed to the back of the box, his head high, the whites of his eyes showing, his body trembling. After a while I was able to step just inside the door but every time I raised my hand his behaviour became violent. So I decided to use the pony's owner as a surrogate to give the healing, something fortunately I rarely have to do. Standing next to Jackie I placed my hand on her back and asked her to hold her hand out to the pony and let him nuzzle it. After a while he calmed down and started to take quick stabs at Jackie's hand. As he made a contact I concentrated on sending healing through her to Theo. Jackie suddenly said, 'Oh, I've got a funny feeling in my tummy and my hand has gone really hot and heavy.' Theo's head started to droop, his eyelids flickered, he sighed. The healing was having an effect. The little pony started to sway as his back softened and his neck lengthened.

As the healing took effect and the barriers came down Theo communicated what had caused his shock. Some men had got into his field and beat him over the head and body and tried to put a rope around his neck. They had wanted to steal him and had been disturbed. (I should point out that at this stage I had been told nothing at all about the pony. It was afterwards that Jackie filled me in with the details and it all fitted together.) At the end of the healing Theo looked very sleepy so we shut the stable door and went and had a coffee. Two days later I saw the vet who had referred me to this case and said she had a big hug for me from the owner. Apparently, after I left, Jackie decided to go back to the stables and opening the door she had a strong feeling that something was different, something had changed. Both ponies were lying down and the air, she said, was thick with a heavy peacefulness. On impulse she took the head collar and approached Theo. He did not flinch away, he remained still as Jackie slipped it around his head – for the first time in eight months. She said afterwards to me it was as if the whole terrible eight months hadn't happened and she suddenly had her pony back.

I visited again the following week and was very pleased to see a much calmer and happier pony. On the second visit Theo let me touch him and I was able to do a full healing treatment all over his body. Again I got a very good response and the pony was very relaxed at the end, sighing and rocking from side to side. His skin was much softer and looser than before the treatment started and on this occasion also he lay down and had a sleep after his healing. He was altogether quite unrecognisable from the pony I had first met and is now a very happy little chap again.

Henry's antisocial behaviour

Henry is a horse who'd had a complete breakdown as a result of his treatment by people. When I first saw him it was an icy January day and he was standing in the middle of a four-acre field, rigid with tension and stress.

> She said afterwards to me it was as if the whole terrible eight months hadn't happened and she suddenly had her pony back.

> If I raised my hands he moved away so I dropped them and concentrated on sending healing across the space between us.

Henry, who was seven at the time, hadn't been caught for five months and was due to be re-backed by natural horse methods in the spring but he needed some help before then to erase his awful memories. He had been with his present owners for eight months, having spent two days travelling on a boat and a lorry without food or water, arriving badly dehydrated. He had been bred in Argentina as a polo pony so had, as a five-year-old, already made a long journey to the dealer who eventually sent him to England. A natural trainer had been called in and for a while the horse had submitted to being caught and handled. He had played some polo and was ridden out but as soon as he was turned away for the winter he'd gone back to square one, the stress syndrome returning. His training had not held because he was too emotionally disturbed and he was antisocial and nervous – and he hated people.

I decided to go into the field and see how close I could get to give him healing. I could get to within 20 feet before he turned his back and moved off, so this was his comfort zone. If I raised my hands he moved away so I dropped them and concentrated on sending healing across the space between us. Henry communicated many beatings, especially around the head, and being left with a sack over his head, and he had a sore back. He watched me suspiciously but after about five minutes I saw the tell-tale signs of endorphin release – the healing was getting through. His head started to drop and his eyes flickered and momentarily shut, his whole body lengthened. Then he started to sway, once or twice buckling at the knee, and he became smaller as tension left him. One of his owners, who had been standing next to me, was suddenly affected by the healing energy that I was sending across to the horse and she left the field to sit down. After a while Henry began to lick and chew in acceptance and he let out a long sigh. That was enough for that day.

When I returned, to my delight I found a much more relaxed Henry in a small corral standing by the gate. His owners said that the very same day after my last visit he began calling to them and became friendlier. He would approach them and take feed calmly as they held a bucket. On this occasion I could stand about eight feet away and I was able to raise my hands to point them at Henry but he would not let me touch him. He responded in the same way as the first treatment and was noticeably calmer when I left. I saw him once more before the trainer came and he was unrecognisable from my first visit. His body shape had changed from stiff and tense to rounded and soft. He was friendly towards his owners and enjoyed their company – he had found peace.

After Henry had been re-schooled I went back and did two treatments where I was able to touch him all over his body. On both of these occasions he began to shake all during the healing over even though he remained relaxed. This is quite a rare reaction but was because he is so sensitive to the changes in energy (this is something that I also get occasionally in people). Henry had the physiotherapist to treat his back and check his saddle and is now successfully used as a polo pony. He is still quite highly strung but he has not reverted to any disturbed behaviour and is easy to handle.

Milly's apprehension

I had offered my services to an equine rescue centre and the first time I visited I was due to treat five of the neediest cases. The stables at the centre are situated under cover in a huge barn building and rather than go into the horses' stables I chose a large quiet area to one side. There were two reasons for this: one was the large number of people that day who wanted to watch me work, but more important was the nervous state of most of the horses. I did not want to invade their safe space and add to their insecurity. I always explain to people that when treating traumatised horses I prefer not to be given many details about them. This is so that my own mind does not interfere with the information that is communicated from the horse.

As we all stood chatting before I started my healing I had noticed the little chestnut horse pressed into the corner at the back of her box. She looked tense and depressed. She took a few steps forward to look over the door and as someone came past she immediately shot to the back of her stable. This was my first patient, Milly, a ten-year-old chestnut mare. Her own special groom went in to get her and as she was led across the corridor towards me every nerve in her body trembled. Her head was up high and she looked wildly from side to side. Fear and apprehension was written all over her face.

Milly eventually stood before me and everything about her said, 'No, I don't want anything to do with humans.' There was absolute quiet as I stepped forward to pick up the horse's emotions. As I stood next to her

I was perplexed to feel absolutely nothing. It was as though the silence in the building had stopped all communication between us. I walked around her several times and stopped in various places to see what I could feel. Again I picked up absolutely nothing. Then after about five minutes as I looked at Milly I realised I was facing a wall – a wall of such pain and misery that the horse had blocked out everything. The silence in the room was a reflection of the silence and numbness inside the horse. I touched Milly softly on her chest, speaking to her and asking her to let me help her.

She turned her head and as our eyes met I saw the wall start to drop and such huge emotion began to pour out of her. The feeling hit me very hard in the centre of the chest and I struggled not to cry. I had to stop for a few seconds and compose myself, so that I was able to continue to help her with healing. As I turned my head slightly I saw that several of the grooms were tearful and sniffing into tissues. They told me afterwards that at that precise moment they had felt her emotional release too and Milly began to sigh with peace. Then I moved my hands from Milly's chest to her neck to begin and as I did so I began to feel as though I was in a fog. It felt like I'd been in this fog for a long time.

I spent about 20 minutes placing my hands in various places on Milly's back and head, places I intuitively felt blockages of energy were being held. As I gave her healing she began to sway softly and gently and her body began to shrink as tension left her. At the end of the healing treatment Milly stood with her head drooping and her body rocking from side to side. Her eyes were shut for a while, the lids trembling. There was a lovely feeling of peace around Milly now and I stood quietly watching her until she came out of her reverie. She reached forward with her head and brushed the back of my hand with her nose – as if to say thank you for helping me.

Milly looked different, relaxed – normal. She was happy to stand there for a while and I discussed her case with the staff. They told me that they'd had the horse for several months and she'd come from a place where she was ill treated. She was considered difficult to handle for various reasons and therefore she was frequently drugged to handle her and also to 'keep her quiet'. She was also left inside on her own for long periods of time. Hence the feeling of fog surrounding me when I was treating her.

Only one groom had been able to approach Milly in all the time that she had been at the rescue centre. The staff had wondered if they would be able to re-house the horse as she was so wary of people, and when prospective owners came she always backed away. Shortly after the healing, Milly slowly followed her groom back to her stable. This time she walked in a very relaxed manner like she didn't have a care in the world. She wandered in to her stable and stood with her head over the door.

We stood discussing the case when suddenly a member of the public wandered in and stopped by Milly's box. The woman stopped, raised her hand and patted the mare's neck. She stood absolutely still and allowed the contact to be made and even nuzzled the woman. One of the staff said, 'That is really amazing, she would normally have bolted to the back of the stable.' So healing for Milly produced an immediate and dramatic change. Within two weeks she had bonded to a kind young lady who visited the centre looking for a horse, and shortly afterwards she went to her new home where she is very settled and very happy.

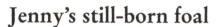

Jenny's still-born foal

GRIEVING ANIMALS

Donkeys always seem to look sad but never have I seen one look as miserable as Jenny. I had gone to a friend's house for supper and during the evening she mentioned that she had a new arrival in her stables at the bottom of the garden. She had been looking for a companion for her pony and had just acquired a donkey. It was not very well, she informed me, in fact the vet was most concerned and had spent quite a bit of time watching over Jenny.

I was off down the garden, unable to eat my dinner until I had given the newcomer some healing. Jenny lay on a thick straw bedding and I thought that she was very ill. Her grief and depression echoed around the stable and lay thick on the balmy evening air. Jenny was not a young donkey, her vet guessed around 25 years old, but just five days earlier she had given birth to a still-born foal. Her new owner had found her traumatised after the birth at a country park and had immediately negotiated to buy her. The donkey's feet were very long, needing urgent attention from the farrier, and one shoulder was deformed, causing some pain. She also had a lot of post-birth discomfort, but it was her profound grief that hung in the air.

I knelt down on the straw next to her and put my hands either side of her neck. She moaned softly and closed her eyes, leant against me and then laid her head across my lap. We stayed like that for a long time, and as I prayed for her to find peace from her suffering I could feel her tears and the mother's love for a child. I put my hands on her back and belly as well and in certain places the areas under them became very hot. After I had finished the healing Jenny stood up and the look in her eyes was softer. She then gave a long yawn as if to let go and I felt hopeful for her recovery.

> I put my hands on her back and belly as well and in certain places the areas under them became very hot.

Before I returned home I went back down to the stables and gave her more healing, with a similar reaction. I gave Jenny's owner some instructions to continue the healing and over the next few days she got good reactions. I returned a week later to find a very different little donkey. Jenny was very bright and cheerful, and doing her version of galloping off round the field. I brought her in to treat her only to see her drop down on her knees and escape under the very low gap left by a bar across the door. Laughing her head off she trotted away saying, 'I'm OK now, thanks.' Jenny has become a much loved family pet and is very sweet natured with everyone, but she continues to escape under, over and through all of the gates, doors and fences.

Knight Errant's life-long friend

Knight Errant was very famous in his day, winning a major championship at Wembley. He is a willing and kind chestnut gelding Anglo-Arab and has been in his present home for over 18 years. His owners called me to see him because stiffness associated with old age was now setting in – the horse was over 21, on medication and beginning to feel a little jaded. For one reason or another it was about three weeks before I could get to see Knight, even though he lived not far from me, but the main problem when I got to see him was not old age but severe grief. Knight had a best friend, a pony called Filly, who he had shared his life with for the past 18 years. Three days before my visit to Knight the pony, aged 33 years, had died in the paddock, a terrible shock for everyone.

Knight was running up and down the fence calling for his friend when I arrived then he went and stood by his stable, but at this stage I was not aware of what had happened. The first thing that I picked up from Knight was his communication that, 'It used to be so different, then everything changed.' He felt he couldn't cope, it had been one thing after the other and now a huge sense of loss. I conveyed all this to Knight's owners who then told me about the death of his friend and it all fell into place.

I placed my hand gently on to the left side of the horse's neck and started tuning in to give him much-needed healing and he was immediately very responsive, becoming very still. When I started to treat him he was stiff and holding his head high but within about three minutes his head started to drop, inch by inch, until his nose touched the ground. Gradually he began to let go, his head flicking as he released the negative energy of his grief and loss. At this stage both owners started to feel things themselves as the energy changed in and around the horse. One felt wobbly in his legs and the hand holding the lead rope was tingly. The other owner felt a strange pulse in his finger tips and then felt very tired. At the end of the treatment Knight gave a long sigh and a couple of big yawns. He looked much more peaceful and relaxed.

At the end of the treatment Knight gave a long sigh and a couple of big yawns.

I visited Knight again a short while later and his owners reported that the healing had definitely helped him. After I had left he didn't call for his friend again and the following day he was more like his old self, friendlier and calmer. He also began to eat better and was generally brighter. Knight is retired with a new companion now but of course things will never be quite the same for him. Healing at the time of his grief definitely helped him to get over the worst of his terrible loss.

Michael's aches and pains

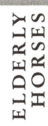

Michael is a much-loved 20-year-old grey Arab horse who I was asked to visit by his owner Monika. He has all the stamp of his breed, a finely chiselled head and an intelligent eye. Michael had suffered much discomfort in his life from long-standing foot and back problems and also several unfortunate accidents. Over the years Monika had lavished a lot of attention, care and expense on the horse and he'd had lots of physiotherapy to help him stay supple. Monika was very upset as she had come to the conclusion that Michael would have to be put to sleep very soon as he appeared so miserable. She felt she couldn't cope without him in her life, and her dearest wish was to move him from the livery yard to her home when building works were complete.

When I first went to see Michael he was lame and on medication from the vet to help kill the pain, and he certainly looked unhappy and in low spirits – so much so that a vet had described him as looking as though he had just left a war zone. Michael stood in the stable with his neck rigid and any steps he took were faltering. I quickly picked up that the horse had a headache, felt uncomfortable in his jaw and ached all over. He communicated that he felt depressed at the months of pain he'd had and wished he could break through and lead a normal life again. He also said quite clearly that he wasn't ready to give up yet. Michael was very responsive to the healing and he stood very quietly while I treated him as he became deeply relaxed. His energy level did feel very weak when I started but I felt a better flow quite quickly. Monika was very emotional throughout the treatment but as it proceeded she said she was starting to feel lighter and Michael got more and more perky. At the end he was much livelier and I explained that healing would have released endorphins to give natural pain relief and re-energised the horse.

I went back two weeks later and was very pleased to see an improved and sound Michael being led in from the field. Monika said she had been able to ride him again as he was so much better. In fact, he was feeling so well that he was spooking and looking for fun. Michael's neck muscles were much less tense, his coat around the chest had a softer feeling and he was putting on weight. Monika commented that the healing had given them a link and better understanding as well as improving her horse's health. 'The healing has given Michael back a sense of wholeness,' she said. During the second treatment, Michael again became very lively and energised. As we walked back to my car he was shouting for his tea and kicking the door. Monika was delighted. I continued to see Michael regularly and six months later Monika realised her dream to take him home. When I saw this gleaming proud horse galloping along the hedgerows of his paddocks, his tail flying high in typical Arab fashion and throwing in a few bucks for good measure, it was a precious reward indeed. You can judge for yourself how well the horse looks now – he is featured on the front cover of the book.

Sally's fits

Horses know much more than we realise and this was a classic example of a wise old horse. Three times in a couple of weeks 24-year-old Sally had collapsed in her field – the vet had checked her out thoroughly but her heart was strong, so epilepsy was suspected and her owner was told she didn't have long to live. Her owner was distraught as she'd had the old horse from a foal and wanted her to be at peace at the end of her life. As I put my hand on her chest Sally told me she was very stressed because she

CASE HISTORIES

felt as though she was on the scrap heap, she wasn't ridden any more and she knew that her owner had a new horse. Sally felt that she was now second best and she felt very low. When I gave this information to the owner she was amazed. Sally had been retired about three months before due to bad arthritis and the owner admitted that she had bought a youngster a month ago – but how did Sally know? The newcomer was deliberately kept several miles away at a livery yard so that the old horse wouldn't be upset at seeing it being handled or ridden. Somehow Sally knew this fact and the stress seemed to have triggered off the fits.

During the treatment I asked the owner to put her hands on the horse's chest as I worked around the body joining both in the healing energy. It was a warm sunny evening and we stood in a beautiful meadow surrounded by woods, golden beams from the late sun dancing through the trees. We seemed to be surrounded in a different type of glow and for a moment the background sounds of the birds and farm animals became muted. Sally stood rock still with her eyes closed and her owner said her arms felt very heavy. Some baby rabbits broke the spell as they ran out from under a bush and chased each other through the wild flowers. The horse's owner was very tearful at the end of the treatment – I had worked hard to let Sally know that she would always be first in her affections and was much loved. If her time on earth was coming to an end she would at least be at peace. When I checked after about a week the horse was very well and the owner said she appeared to have a new lease of life. More than eighteen months later Sally happily lives out her retirement with several horse friends and has not had any more fits.

Sally stood rock still with her eyes closed and her owner said her arms felt very heavy.

Pristina's liver disease

It was a very urgent telephone call that took me to Pristina. A vet had given Alison my details as he thought that I could help both horse and owner in their distress. When I first saw Pristina it was a real shock. I could see that she had been a beautiful, six-year-old, fine-boned chestnut Arab. Now she was very thin and her face was so badly burnt that she looked grotesque, and her legs were swollen and weeping. A child's shirt was tied loosely across her face to help prevent daylight from irritating the skin further and also to keep flies out of the weeping wounds. Pristina was suffering from

TERMINALLY-ILL HORSES

99

the worst photosensitisation reaction I had ever seen. This is something that often happens when there is severe liver damage. Sunlight reacts with the skin to result in terrible burning (and it can happen even on a cloudy day). The horse had suffered mild problems the previous summer but she had recovered well and had been full of beans until she suddenly developed a severe attack of colic and was rushed to an equine hospital for emergency surgery. A gangrenous gut was diagnosed from worm damage, which it was suspected the horse had as a foal. A large section of her intestine was removed during the operation but she made a very good recovery, with no problems until that day in the sun.

In Pristina's short life she'd had six owners but none had loved her as deeply as her present one. As a two-year-old she had been rescued, together with several others, from a person who was the subject of a very high-profile RSPCA prosecution case. Now her loving owner was desperately trying to nurse her back to good health. 'We're the best of mates,' said Alison, who spent nearly every minute of the day helping the horse. When I saw Pristina liver disease was suspected and a vet was due to come back the next day to perform a biopsy. Although very sick, the horse was a fighter and was beginning to respond to the antibiotics but I felt that possibly too much organ damage had been done and that healing was going to help the horse find peace at the end of her life.

I ran my hands over Pristina's sides feeling for places where the energy was most blocked. As I passed over the liver meridians I felt a prickly pulsing in my fingertips and waves of heat rose from her body. I got the same reaction from the spleen area so I gave a lot of healing to these places. Pristina also communicated a headache as a result of liver toxins and shock and I spent a long time placing my hands on strategic points on her head to give as much pain relief as possible. She showed a typical endorphin response – the sign that natural painkillers were being released into the blood stream, one of the benefits of healing. Her owner said that she too felt a lightness come over her as I treated her horse, that a weight fell from her shoulders as the feeling of peace entered her and Pristina too looked much brighter when I left.

I saw Pristina again a few days later – the biopsy result confirmed cirrhosis of the liver with associated ragwort poisoning. The horse's face was healing very well although her legs were still in a bad way. Alison said that although Pristina was ill she seemed more contented and definitely peaceful – she was active and whickering to her a lot and eating very well. The vet had said that the pony might have a chance and put her on to a special diet. Again she was very responsive to healing; in fact, she loved it. Her owner said she looked as though she was in ecstasy.

The third time I visited Pristina, a week later, the legs still had not healed but she looked very perky and her eye was noticeably very bright. In fact, a vet had commented on this very fact just the day before. When I arrived, Pristina rushed to the front of the stable calling to me and pushed her nose into my hands in greeting, licking my fingers. I stood back and took a long look at her – the aura around her looked very weak, the energy field was dark and I felt that she had not much time left. I began to give her healing and as on the previous occasions she became calm and sedated, then suddenly she started to shake and lay down. I asked for the vet to be called who confirmed that the liver had flooded the system with toxins and the time had come to let her go. Pristina was peacefully put to sleep under the arms of the surrounding woodland trees. Although I only knew her a short time she enriched my life with her strength and courage and the abundance of love she had to give.

Smartie's tumour

At first no one knew that Smartie was terminally ill. He was a very handsome thoroughbred eventer, an absolute gentleman of 17 years of age, who had the most wonderful kind manners and was a real schoolmaster. The big horse had suddenly and quickly become very tired and weak and he was whisked off to an equine hospital where a range of tests was run. Blood tests showed that his red cell count was dangerously low and he was put on a drip and given daily injections. Day after day his red cell count was monitored but there was no improvement and he remained at the hospital. The vets were puzzled as to what the problem was and Smartie was eventually diagnosed with internal bleeding. In desperation, after the horse had spent over a week at the hospital, Jo called me and asked if I could visit to give him some healing.

Smartie stepped back politely as I entered his stable at the hospital and I could immediately sense his depletion of energy. He had also become very thin and wasn't eating very much. I laid my hand gently on his side and listened. There was a big energy blockage around the top of the stomach

> Smartie loved the healing treatment and he was a joy to treat, standing very still, rocking in time to the healing rhythm.

area and I also picked up restriction around the throat. Smartie loved the healing treatment and he was a joy to treat, standing very still, rocking in time to the healing rhythm. After the treatment had finished Smartie was noticeably brighter and had perked up. Jo phoned me the next day: the blood test taken after the healing treatment had shown an incredible 50 per cent increase of red blood cells, and the horse had started eating again. I warned Jo not to build up false hopes because healing can produce a tremendous boost but if a serious disease has caused too much tissue damage and deterioration it may not be permanent. Smartie slowly continued to improve, however, and his blood count stabilised. He was definitely brighter and eating better and after a couple more days was sent home, but I was still concerned that there was a very serious problem with him.

I saw Smartie twice more after he got back home. On the first visit his energy field seemed not too bad but it was still weak around the stomach area. As before he responded well to the healing and was very perky afterwards. The next time I went a week later I found the energy flowing through the horse worryingly low, especially in the throat area. This time Smartie was not so revitalised after the healing and stood with his head hanging down. All of a sudden liquid streamed out of his nose for several seconds and a few hours later he started to choke. The vet was called and he was put to sleep by the fields he loved so well. The final diagnosis was a tumour in the oesophagus where it entered the stomach. Healing certainly helped Smartie to be at peace during his illness and gave him an energy boost, which enabled him to spend the last weeks of his life happily at home among the people he loved.

DISTANT HEALING

Twiggy's fear of her rug

I cannot unfortunately be everywhere at once. Also driving long distances is not practical for it is tiring and then I cannot give strong healing treatments. Frequently I am called for help from people who live quite a long way from me and in these cases I arrange to send distant healing to their horses. I ask that the owners send a photograph and a snippet of mane or tail for me to concentrate on and a short covering letter about the problem.

CASE HISTORIES

I have a dedicated healing room at home and most days I spend time sending healing to names on my distant healing list. I sit quietly with meditation music playing softly in the background and concentrate on the individual cases, holding my hand over the photos. By this method I have had some good results for a variety of animals, including horses.

One lady called Georgina called me at her wits' end about her seven-year-old mare Twiggy. Her horse had been fine until one morning when she had found her in a very distressed condition. She was galloping around in the orchard next to her field, having demolished the fence between the two and injuring herself in the process. The previous night she had been turned out in a new, very expensive rug and that had been torn on the fence when she jumped out of her field.

After a few days of rest and attention to her legs Georgina went to put the rug back on Twiggy but the horse worked herself up into a frenzy and began to sweat profusely. When she was put into the field she stood by the gate, obviously distressed and worried. So her owner brought her in and tried another rug – the horse reacted in the same way staying by the gate and refusing to move into the field and graze. Over the months every conceivable reason for Twiggy's reaction to rugs was checked out. The original rug was looked over – it was a soft, lightweight, breathable material and did not crackle. Neither were there any rough edges to irritate the skin. Vets, chiropractors and physiotherapists checked the horse's back and didn't find any pain or stiffness. Trainers tried to school her through the problem but the mare was adamant that she would not have a rug put on her.

They would leave the horse for a few weeks then try again but the mare would panic when any rug was brought near her. If someone got a rug on the horse she would stand fretting in the field by the gate, for hours if necessary, until she was brought in and the rug taken off her, or she would jump out of the field in a very distressed state. Eighteen months went by and the horse went out in all weathers without a rug on, the owner becoming more and more concerned. The phone call to me came just before the start of a winter, and Georgina said to me, 'I just can't bear the thought of Twiggy being cold and wet. If it's a bad winter this year I will be so worried about her.'

I asked Georgina to let me send distant healing for a week to Twiggy and she sent me a photograph to help me focus. Then she was to try on the same rug with which the horse had been found distressed. During the time

I was sending the healing I had the impression that Twiggy had been attacked in her field and someone had grabbed hold of the neck part of the rug, twisting it around her throat. I felt it was a sheer coincidence that the rug was new that night. Georgina confirmed that what I picked up made sense – she had forgotten to tell me that whenever someone went to fasten the buckles across the horse's chest was when she reacted most strongly, rearing up, shaking and sweating.

During the distant healing I concentrated on removing the emotional blockages from Twiggy and sending her some peace of mind. The appointed time came and the next day I received a phone call. Georgina was thrilled and excited to report all had gone well. The previous evening she had put the rug on Twiggy without any problems and had led the horse to her paddock, released her and closed the gate. She couldn't believe her eyes when Twiggy put her head down to graze and began to walk away calmly. She expected the horse to bolt back to the gate any minute but she didn't, so Georgina went off, wondering what she would find on her return. When she came back the next morning she found Twiggy still munching away happily in the middle of the field and from that day on the horse has not had any problem with her rugs.

Sport's sluggishness

Sport is, as his name suggests, a warmblood sport horse. Although a gelding he has all the presence of a stallion. His owner is an instructor and competitor and uses him for a bit of everything, including show jumping, dressage and eventing. He is a very active horse with lots of get up and go, so one morning when he stood quietly in his stable his owner knew that he wasn't well. A couple of days before Sport had competed at a large equestrian centre and the vet suspected that he'd picked up a bug there, and antibiotics were prescribed. Sure enough a day or so later the horse developed a cough and runny nose and was clearly very miserable. After the second course of antibiotics and blood tests the vet said that Sport was OK and to slowly bring him back into work, but the black horse was not his usual boisterous self and was dull and sluggish.

Despite having several weeks' rest Sport was still off colour and it was at this point that I received a call to put him on to my distant healing list. It was just before I sat down to send out the healing so within half an hour of the call I concentrated on Sport. Next morning there was a message for me from the owner: 'Fantastic, keep up the good work, Sport's a lot better. I rode him this morning and he's like his old self.' I carried on sending Sport distant healing for a week, then took him off my list but that day Sport's owner rang to ask me if I'd stopped sending healing to him because he was off-colour again. The horse obviously needed more healing so I sent distant healing for another week. By that time he had fully recovered and was doing well in his work and his owner was very pleased to see him charging round the fields sending the turf flying as he went. Sport is still in good health and enjoys going to competitions again; he certainly has his sparkle and his zest for life back.

By that time he had fully recovered and was doing well in his work and his owner was very pleased to see him charging round the fields sending the turf flying as he went.

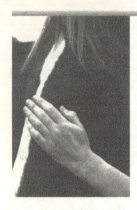

6
How to give a healing treatment

*'A person must be converted twice –
once from the natural to the spiritual
and then again from the spiritual to the natural'*

Eberhard Arnold

The two questions I am most frequently asked by my clients are, 'What can I do to help my horse?' and, 'Can anyone give healing?' My answer to the second question is – yes, with the right attitude and with practice, and then the answer to the first question follows. For by giving healing to the horse, you are helping it. From the need to give healing to horses and clients wishing to help themselves came the idea for this book – to bring the subject of hands-on healing and how to give a treatment to horses to a wider audience. The vital force flows through every living being, through humans and through horses, and gives us a common ground for communication and a means of helping on a level which we may have not previously considered possible.

Sometimes people then say to me, 'But what if I can't give healing to my horse? What if I can't do it?' Well, the healing energy is there for everyone to access and you will never know whether you are gifted in this area if you don't try. Healing is there for everyone to take and give, and some people will be gifted as healers just as people are gifted in other areas. Some people will find it easier than others and will more readily adapt to the subtle information received during a healing session. The gift of healing comes not from the healer but from a higher source in the universe and the healer is a channel for this source. With healing you cannot do any harm but you can do a great deal of good and your horse needs you to help it. So attune to the help which is already there, all around you, just waiting for you to tap into it. It is true that not everyone will be able to take the healing as far or as deep

HOW TO GIVE A HEALING TREATMENT

as it can go because people differ in their ability to work with this energy, feel it, understand, harness and organise it. If you don't try you won't know how much potential you have. If you do you may be pleasantly surprised. If it is not a skill that you develop very strongly then there are always the developed and registered healers to call upon to help your horse.

The following guidelines are intended for use only on your own horses. To practise as a professional animal healer and become a member of an association, an individual needs to join a recognised organisation with the relevant insurance. It is also some guarantee to members of the public that a code of conduct is being followed. Working on members of the public's horses requires more extensive knowledge of the concept of healing and a very strong ability to channel energy. If you have never done so you should go to a healer yourself to experience what it can feel like for your horse. Try to find someone by recommendation; as with anything in life people have individual personalities and styles and some therapists are more gifted than others. Don't be afraid to talk to the healer at length in person or on the telephone and if you feel uneasy about their manner or philosophy move on. You need a rapport with your healer and there is someone out there to suit everyone.

Where possible, incorporating the use of complementary healthcare and remedies into our healing lives is a good idea because they treat us holistically and don't have the side effects that many medications have.

A new journey for you and your horse

Healing is the beginning of a new journey in life. It is something that you will not do just once if you wish to develop your healing potential and it is something that needs to become incorporated into your life. To access the healing we need compassion, as without it healing cannot filter through. Once we open our hearts and minds to healing it allows subtle changes to take place as we become more receptive. Healing becomes part of the fabric of our lives and enables both the human and the horse to find inner peace.

At the beginning don't rush off and try to give healing to all the horses in your yard because you will become disillusioned and fatigued. Choose one horse to spend half an hour with per week for a month and then as you progress try healing on other horses. Starting on a healing pathway is like anything new in life – it takes dedication, practice and especially patience. As you develop your healing potential you will experience different levels of understanding and awareness – it is a very special journey.

Horses are our teachers to teach us skills on a deeper level, and they are wonderful teachers of healing. Horses are also in our lives to teach us responsibility, to teach us to listen, to teach us sensitivity and to teach us to follow our intuition regarding the horse. This intuition is the healing communication from the horse heard by our soul and waiting to be acknowledged. If we can do all these things with the horse we have taken a step forward, for and with mankind, and we will be truly much more in tune with life. Healing horses helps us along our own pathway in life and helps to open up the channels of our intuition.

Setting aside healing time

Choose a time for giving healing to your horse when you will not be rushed or stressed; 20–30 minutes or so is a reasonable time to begin with as any longer can be tiring initially due to the concentration that is required. To really get within the horse and make a change, the focus and intent must be very powerful, and it is this concentration that can be tiring not the healing energy transmitted, for we do not give of our own energy. If you are a tense type of person allow a little more time for it may take you a while to tune in and relax. At the end of a healing session allow yourself a few minutes to absorb the subtle changes and anything you and your horse have experienced together. Then have a glass of water or herbal tea and relax for a while.

Essential things to do during a healing session

❖ Switch off mobile phones and radios.
❖ Ask other people not to come and chat to you or watch you (as you become confident, you may be happy with an audience but it can be distracting at first).
❖ Make sure you are not expecting a delivery or visitors.
❖ Choose a time when a ride is not about to come in or go out of the yard.
❖ Don't break your horse's routine to give healing. If the horse is waiting to be fed or to go out it won't be very relaxed.
❖ Remove any items containing magnets from about yourself or your horse.

HOW TO GIVE A HEALING TREATMENT

When not to give healing

There are some times when a person should not give healing and these include:

- When under the influence of alcohol. In my experience horses dislike the energy from such people anyway and if a person has been drinking their mind is not clear for focusing on or concentrating on healing.
- When under the influence of mind-affecting drugs or medication, for the same reasons.
- During times of extreme stress – for healing channels to be open a healer needs to be calm.
- During times of poor health and illness – the healer's own energy field will be weak and a strong channel will not be formed.
- During times of fatigue and tiredness, for the same reasons.
- When depressed – such negative energy around the horse is unsettling and healing will not be accepted.

Starting the treatment

I always insist that a horse is on a head collar (halter) and lead rope during a healing treatment, with the owner or rider holding the horse as it is a shared experience. With your own horse you may wish to treat it while it is free in a stable (box or stall) or you may wish to have it loosely tied up. If you have a new or nervous horse it is much better and safer if you can get someone to hold it on a rope while you give the healing. Stand quietly by the horse's side near to the head and neck. Keep your hands still then very gently, with one hand, touch the horse on the neck at the brachial major chakra (see Chapter 7). However, you can give healing by laying your hand anywhere on the horse that is comfortable for both of you. There are many places on the horse's body where healing can be channelled. These may or may not correspond with acupuncture points, meridians or chakras.

Imagine that your hand is a butterfly that has gently landed on to the horse's skin and then open your heart and feel love, letting it flow. When

HEALING FOR HORSES

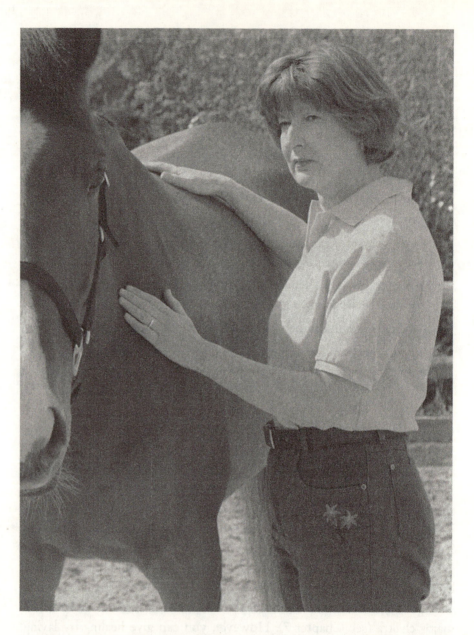

This is usually where I place my hands to begin a healing treatment.

love flows from deep in the soul the healing can be most readily accessed. At this stage it is important that you ask the horse's permission to let the healing through. So much of what we do to horses is a form of assault, because we just barge in and get on with things without any respect for the horse's space or mood. So ask, and it can be out loud or silently through the mind. I say something in my mind like, 'Can I help you to be at peace,

HOW TO GIVE A HEALING TREATMENT

to feel my love and the love from God?' Mostly it is then OK to proceed, but if the horse appears too agitated, try settling it with a small feed and give the healing while it is eating (it doesn't affect the treatment adversely). If this doesn't work, try another time or give distant healing. Generally it is best to change the idea that humans can do anything they wish to any other creature, and by asking permission to give healing, by *offering* healing, we open up another level of understanding and communication with the horse.

Let your love flow into the horse's mind and ask permission from the horse to help him or her. Put all negative thoughts out of your mind. These can influence healing energy – instead concentrate on sending out thoughts of love, harmony and peace. Be unselfish with your reasons for giving the healing.

At the end of giving healing take a moment or two to thank the healing source for working with you and your horse – it doesn't matter where you personally think that source is or what you think it is.

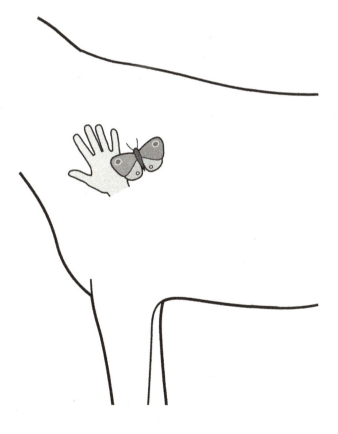

Use a very light touch for giving healing. Imagine that your hand is a butterfly landing on the horse.

HEALING FOR HORSES

Where to place your hands

❖ Using points from the charts here and on page 132 as guidance, place your hands lightly on or over these areas. Be careful not to apply any pressure – your hand should be as gentle as a butterfly.

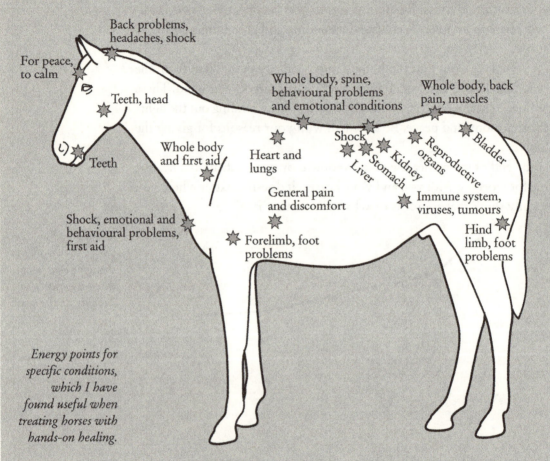

Energy points for specific conditions, which I have found useful when treating horses with hands-on healing.

❖ Don't wave your hands around over the horse or move them quickly on the body – keep them as still as possible and don't fidget. When you move your hands move them very slowly and gently. Speak to the horse softly and tell it what you are doing. This is important because otherwise you can disturb and ruffle the horse's aura and you will find the horse will probably get agitated and even cross. Then the healing will not be accepted.

HOW TO GIVE A HEALING
TREATMENT

❖ Hands-on healing requires the giver to link the healing energy to the horse so that the horse can take what it needs. We should never force it or try to decide where it should go. Where we think the source of the problem lies is not always the right place for the healing to go to.

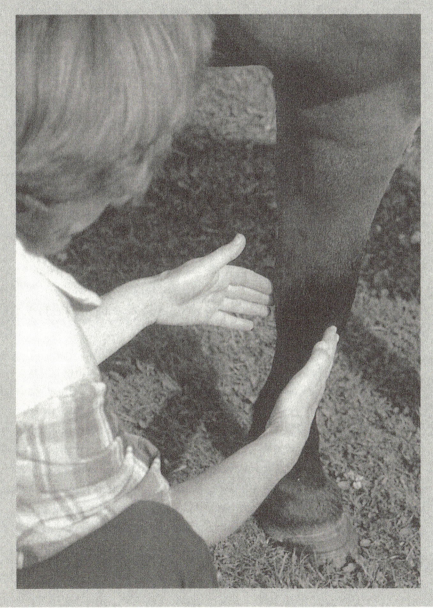

Use the fingers of one or both hands to point and direct healing energy to specific areas of injury. Energy flows in pulses from the finger tips.

Working intuitively

As you progress and become more confident about what you are feeling and the results you are getting you can try working intuitively. You can use your hands as a dowsing instrument. Hold your hands slightly above the horse's body. As you pick up areas of energy blockage you may feel hot spots, cold spots, tingling or pulsing under your hands. When you find these spots keep your hands over this place until the areas underneath them change.

You are using your hands like a magnet to release the congestion from

Keep it simple

Life today is increasingly hectic and demanding and mankind seeks to invent ever more complicated methods of trying to redress the balance. Individuals and companies stand to make a great deal of money from re-inventing the wheel or trying to create a magic potion to solve both our own and our horses' problems. We have lost sight of many of the answers because we make everything more intricate, yet healing is simple and literally at our fingertips. In my previous career, when I worked in marketing, there were lots of systems and formulas to follow but one of these is actually useful in explaining how to use healing. It's called KISS, which means 'keep it simple'.

When we seek to overcomplicate and confuse things, including healing, KISS is a good thing to remember. When beginning to give healing to horses, or any living being for that matter, just allow yourself to be natural and uncomplicated. Both you and your horse will enjoy it more and you actually have everything you need to succeed – your love, your compassion and your touch. The simpler the approach to healing, the more effective it will be. The divine spark is in each one of us and we can let it be a bright light or an extinguished flame, as we so choose. You will develop your own style and way of working that is part of your understanding according to your sensitivity, which is something that I have done over the years. As you become more in tune with the healing forces and your inner self, this sensitivity and your awareness expand.

the electromagnetic field of the horse. Check this area again the next time you give healing to the horse. If the same area keeps getting congested consider what may be happening and whether there are any early warning health signs. Is the saddle to blame or the bridle? Has the horse been injured, is he unusually tense, depressed or off colour? Have you noticed changes in behaviour? Carry on giving regular healing but consider asking the vet to examine the horse and give a diagnosis.

Tuning in

Your intent is very important and is your link with the healing energy. As you stand with your hand on the horse the intention in your mind and the love in your heart must be quite clear if you wish to help the horse on a mental, emotional and physical level. Focus on this intention as strongly as you possibly can, pushing all other thoughts out of your mind. Thoughts have a very powerful energy all of their own and many healers can encourage big energy movements and changes in a living being by transferring energy which has a root in a strong wish to help. It is very important to keep negativity out of the mind (and body) when giving healing to the horse – negativity is the creator of a closed mind and for effective healing your mind needs to be open. It sounds very complicated but it's not once you get the hang of it. Just go out and relax and it will come together.

During the healing treatment, then, relax and have an open mind. Unless you are giving healing to the site of a specific injury or wound, don't direct your thoughts to where you think the healing should go. Energy follows the thought pattern – the intent – and if you have focused on one particular aspect of the horse or one particular place it may not be the right place, or not the only place where there is a blockage. Open your mind and ask for the healing energy to go to wherever it is needed, on whatever level, and wait for some sign that healing is beginning to come through. Watch the horse's face for a surprised expression, a flicker of the eyes, a drop of the head. Then you are ready to move on to the other points that you wish to work over. If you do not get a reaction initially do not give up, carry on and complete the treatment. It will always have some effect, providing you keep that intent to heal in your mind. It takes time to build up the lines of healing communication and, of course, some people will be much more adept at this than others, as with anything in life. But remember, everyone has access to healing energy.

The horse's comfort during healing

During cold or chilly weather do not take your horse's rugs off to give healing. It is unfair for the horse to be allowed to get cold and unnecessary tension is stressful and can make the healing less effective. After all, when healers treat people they do not ask them to strip clothes off but place their hands over the patient's clothes. It is the same with horses and rugs, the

Your horse must always be comfortable when you give healing. During cold or chilly weather do not take your horse's rugs off to give a treatment. Healing energy travels through the material, which is just a mass of energy units anyway.

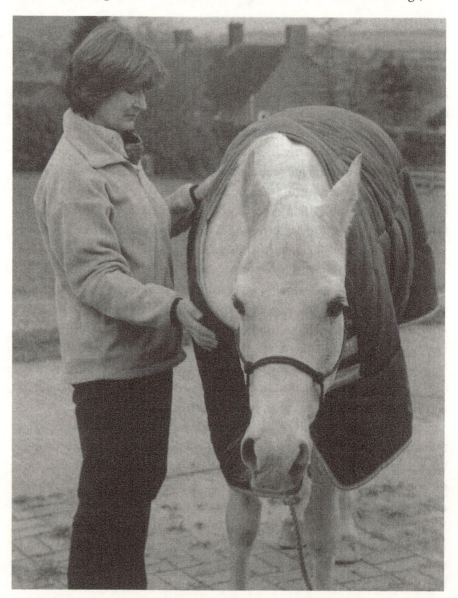

HOW TO GIVE A HEALING TREATMENT

healing energy travels through them as material itself is just a mass of energy units anyway.

Choose a quiet restful place to give healing to the horse, where there is a nice deep bed. Concrete is not good for horses' legs or backs and not comfortable for horses to stand on. Give healing within the horse's normal routine so that it is as relaxed as possible. If you go for a healing treatment yourself your practitioner will make sure that you are comfortable on a couch or in a chair so that you can relax and it's only fair to treat our equines the same way. If a horse is standing in a draughty corridor, on a hard concrete floor or in a busy thoroughfare it is not conducive to what we are trying to achieve. Also if a horse needs friends nearby then it is a good idea to bring a companion in as well to keep stress levels down during the healing.

Young horses

Treating young horses is like giving healing to babies and children: can be fidgety and easily distracted. I therefore always keep the treatment times

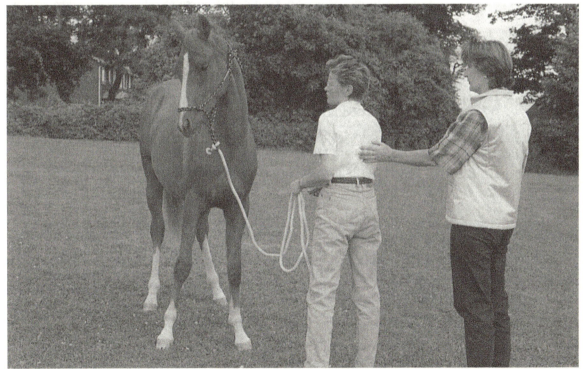

Giving healing to a young and nervous Arab colt, Edward, using the owner as a surrogate to channel the healing energy through (see page 90).

to a minimum as there is absolutely no point in setting up a stressful situation or confrontation. Foals and young horses, like most children, I find are very receptive anyway to healing so a lot can be achieved in a short time. Remember that healing, energy can travel into the body very quickly. Little and often is the key here and it is important not to chastise fidgety behaviour. Nervous horses should be treated in the same way during a healing session.

The reactions you can expect from the horse

Given below is a list of the reactions I have noticed in horses from healing treatments that I have given over the years. In some horses I have noted all of these responses, in others a few. During my healing sessions on horses I have found that the greatest percentage become very calm and sedated during the sessions. A smaller number become agitated, apparently due to their being worried by the tingly feeling during the healing and I may have to reduce the treatment time because of this. This does not, however, affect how successful the treatment can be. Only a split second of relaxation is needed to allow the energy field of the horse to rebalance and strengthen. Light from the sun travels to the earth in less than ten minutes, which shows how fast energy can move. In this smaller group I have noticed that they frequently include the following types of horses:

- Horses with sensitive skins, itchy skins.
- Easily worried horses.
- Those with a short attention span.
- Those with very tense owners.
- Horses with a past history of physical or mental abuse.

The reactions you can expect from the horse

- Endorphin effect – the horse becomes sleepy, eyes close, head droops and nods.
- Nostrils quiver, whiskers quiver.
- The mouth becomes saggy, tension eases.
- Wrinkles around the eyes smooth out.

HOW TO GIVE A HEALING
TREATMENT

- ❖ Ears flick half back to listen to what's going on in the body – a sign of attention to and acceptance of the healing.
- ❖ Head raises and the horse appears to be looking back along its body.
- ❖ The horse paws at the ground or stomps the ground. It may be unusual for that particular horse to do so.

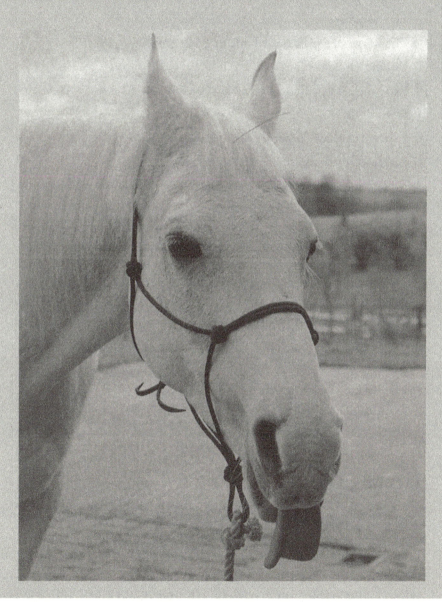

Horses are usually very relaxed and peaceful during a healing treatment. Signs of the deep inner peace include sighing, yawning, licking and chewing. The facial muscles relax – lips and nostrils become droopy and quiver. Ears are pointed towards the body listening to the sensations from the healer's hands.

119

- The horse becomes itchy and wants to nibble at the skin.
- The horse becomes unsteady on its legs.
- The horse sways from side to side.
- Muscle twitches (kinetic releases of energy).
- The tail jerks up and stretches out.
- The horse arches its neck and stretches back.
- The horse stretches out of one or both hind legs.
- Licking and chewing.
- Snorting and clearing airways.
- Deep sighs.
- Change in skin temperature in various places.
- Increased or decreased respiratory rate.
- Nudging owner – attention-seeking to say, 'Look what's happening to me.'
- Skin changes – the skin is the largest organ of the body and the most visible. It is a good gauge therefore of the relaxation benefits of healing. Brands may stand out more and the skin around the neck and shoulders can be softer and looser. There may be an added lustre to the coat. Often clients have noticed skin changes on their horses after a healing treatment.
- Yawning.
- Vocal noises.
- The back drops and becomes very relaxed.
- Shivering.

Healing time

After the treatment your horse will go into healing time and may be a bit sleepy, and as you get more proficient at giving healing the after effects should become more noticeable. I always allow the horse to rest and come out of the sleepiness naturally and request that horses are worked or ridden before healing on the day of a treatment, not afterwards. No harm

HOW TO GIVE A HEALING TREATMENT

would come to the horse but the reason is to allow the horse the chance to absorb the beneficial changes and to feel the deep peace and inner relaxation. Sudden and acute stress can cancel out healing benefits as the rush of adrenaline increases cellular activity.

Also it is advisable not to have the farrier or other therapists arrive a short while after healing for the same reasons. Some quite big changes can take place during the first session so it's important for the horse to rest afterwards. Exceptions to this are competition horses where healing can be beneficial during an event or show, and healing given as first aid.

How many treatments are necessary to help the horse?

If the horse has a chronic problem then healing can be given regularly, every few days. For sudden acute problems or long periods of confinement due to illness or injury then I would recommend giving a healing treatment to your horse every day.

Unusual currents and pulses flow through the horse's body when healing is given and the horse needs time to absorb the changes, which stimulate repair or rebalancing on whatever level is possible. Sometimes healing is successful in one session, more often results are progressive and appear over a period of time.

Healing as first aid

With both humans and animals I have been able to give healing effectively as first aid and if your horse suddenly falls ill or is injured this is something that you can do while waiting for the veterinary surgeon to arrive. Don't be surprised if at this time you feel something strange under your hands, as the energy field of the horse will be spinning out of balance. Just keep your hand on the horse and focus your mind on the healing. I have shown some points on the chart as to where it is beneficial to give first aid healing (see page 112), but you can touch the horse anywhere for the healing to enter.

If the horse is too upset to be touched or it is too dangerous then stand back and hold out your hand, pointing your fingers at the stricken animal. Allow your mind to stay strong and imagine rays of light pouring from your finger tips. The horse will feel this healing energy and be comforted. The sooner healing is given after an accident or injury the better. Lay your hands on the horse to give healing for it to help on all levels; don't treat symptoms such as an injury or wound until after the vet has attended to them. Then you can treat individual areas with healing as well as focusing on general healing – emotionally and mentally as well as physically.

Some of the things the horse can feel during treatments

Horses can be expected to feel one or more of the things outlined below – initially they will feel a tingling as the healing stimulates the electromagnetic field. It is at this stage that a small number of horses start to get agitated or worried. Most settle down once they realise that it's going to be OK but a minority panic and then I would recommend a shorter

What the horse can feel during healing

- Tingling in a part of the body or throughout the whole body.
- Being light-headed.
- Heaviness in one or more limbs.
- Heat in a part of the body or throughout all the body.
- Shivery.
- Intermittent temperature changes.
- Twinges throughout the body.
- Unusual pulses in parts of the body.
- Emotional upsets or tearfulness. Horses, of course, do not cry but they feel the same emotion and disturbed energy, which in humans we release as tears.
- Increased or decreased breathing rate.
- Drifting, mind wandering.
- Sleepiness, great tiredness.

treatment, perhaps use the owner as a surrogate or even treat from a distance. It only needs a split second of a deep reaction for the beneficial changes to activate.

The horse feels a great many things during healing. How do I know this? From three sets of information:

❖ Because nearly always during treatments bystanders will tell me of things that are happening to them, which I know is a reflection of what is happening to the horse.

❖ By the horse's reaction during healing it is obvious that it is feeling something unusual.

❖ From the feedback from humans who have had healing. Horses' bodies are comprised of blood, flesh, bone and nerve endings the same as ours and they can physically feel what we feel – and maybe more.

What the healer can feel when giving treatment to the horse

The healer needs to be in control of the energy in that you don't actually want to be feeling too much too strongly otherwise it can be tiring. The place to get the strongest sensation is within the mind because then you are operating on the highest level. If the healer becomes physically light-headed or wobbly then he or she is not in a safe position to be treating the horse. I advise that if anyone experiences any of these sensations during the treatment they should stop, step back, ask their body to clear it away and start again. Commonly healers may feel heat in their hands or tingling and that is perfectly all right to work with. I feel that any other sensations should be guarded against and the key is to be in control of the healing energy, not to let it control you – the ultimate aim, after all, is healing for the horse.

Some people may not feel anything in their hands while giving healing to their horse, but if you can see a beneficial effect for the horse then do not worry unduly about this, it just happens sometimes. As you develop you should become more intuitive as your horse communicates to you what it needs. You are now beginning to hear him – your healing journey is taking you down a path of wonderful discovery and adventure.

Sensations a healer may feel with horses

- Heat under the hands and fingers or in the palm.
- Tingling in the fingers.
- Hot or cold spots on the body of the horse.
- Pulsing in the fingertips or hands.

Conditions where hands-on healing can help horses

Healing today works on problems with a root cause frequently based in yesterday. Healing can help with any condition because it is the basis of homeostasis (balance in the body) and can work on an emotional, mental or physical level. Here is a list of the most frequent reasons why I have been asked to give healing to horses and there have been some good results. However, you can give healing to your horse for anything you feel the need for. Even if you feel all is well give healing anyway just because you love your horse.

- Grief
- Change of home/owner
- Previous ill treatment (no matter how long ago)
- Emotional/behavioural problems
- Depression
- Post-viral syndrome
- Injuries and accidents
- After surgery
- Pain relief
- Inflammation
- Tumours
- Liver problems
- General illness
- Pregnancy
- Problems in foals
- Old age
- Terminal illness
- Arthritis
- Shock
- Headaches
- Low immune system

Remember that healing works by treating the horse holistically, which means it doesn't treat symptoms but the whole horse. By treating the horse at a deep level individual problems may resolve themselves.

Always call a vet first if your horse has a problem of *any kind*, a delay could result in something serious.

Treating the terminally-ill horse

The feeling of peace that healing can give to the terminally ill horse is priceless. Hands-on healing releases endorphins from the brain into the blood stream and they have an opiate-like effect, bringing natural pain relief and a feeling of improved wellbeing. Healing to this horse can be given daily, even twice daily and certainly just before the vet's final visit. You will be feeling upset and emotional during this time but carry on placing your hands on the horse whenever possible and giving healing, for no matter how short a time. Keep the horse in your thoughts as well. You will help your horse to make the transition to a higher life and will make its spiritual journey easier too. The horse will sense that you are offering healing support in the final hour of need and it will be greatly comforted. This is healing at its most precious, the healing of the mind and spirit for the final journey. You should also find that it leaves you with a sense of calmness as the healing will join you both in another dimension, and you will know that you said goodbye having done everything you could for your friend. After your horse has passed away keep sending out healing thoughts: they will still be received by your horse, for remember, its life force still exists somewhere. Your horse still links with you.

What healing can't do

Healing treatments may not be lasting if the horse is upset because it is lonely or spends too much time in its stable (for the horse it can feel like a prison). Healing won't mend a sore back if the saddle doesn't fit, a sore mouth if the bridle is wrong or the teeth are neglected, or painful feet if the shoeing is inadequate. Initially such a horse can appear happier after healing but after a day or two the stress and pain will unbalance the system again. The owner needs to ask honestly whether there are any improvements to be made and these issues need to be addressed as well as healing being given.

It is a good idea to give healing to the horse after lifestyle improvements are made because due to previous problems the horse can hold on to inner resentment or anger, and healing helps clear away these negative emotions. Inner emotional blockages may later on lead to, or manifest as, behavioural problems or disease. I have frequently treated horses where this type of negative energy had a root cause going back many years and after healing the animal was much happier, showing an improved sense of wellbeing.

Healing won't change a cob into a race horse

Healing isn't going to change the horse's fundamental personality. For example, a shy horse will remain so and a dominant horse will stay leader of the pack. But healing aims to bring out the best and more positive aspects, producing a feeling of inner peace. For this reason, horses have often become much happier and easier to be with after I've treated them, and have done better in their work. Healing isn't going to make a cob into a race horse or an ageing hack into a champion dressage horse – it will help the person inside that horse's body to get in touch with him- or herself and hopefully have a better relationship with humans. Healing can help the horse to realise its potential to the best of its ability and can stimulate repair of cells if needed.

Healing is not a magic wand

Do not expect overnight results with chronic and long-term conditions. Let's keep our feet on the ground. Dramatic and sudden changes ('miracles') can and do happen; however, more often, possible improvements usually show over a period of time. I remember being asked to give healing to a young competition horse which had been lame for a year after a bad fall at speed over a jump. The horse had been seen by vets, chiropractors and an acupuncturist but no one could identify the source of the problem. I quickly laid my hand over pathways in the spine where I noticed energy blockages and felt very sluggish and depleted energy movement and flow (suggesting a serious injury as this affects messages to the limbs).

The horse was very responsive to healing and sleepy for a long time afterwards. He was relieved to let go of his emotional unhappiness as he had spent many months being incarcerated in a stable to see if that would help his problem. At the end of the healing the yard manager asked if they could gallop the horse the next day. I thought they were joking but nevertheless explained why that was impossible. However, they telephoned two days later to say the healing had not worked because the horse was still lame. They did say though that the horse was much easier to handle and brighter, so from my point of view the healing had been successful. We need to be realistic and understand what healing can and can't do – what it is and what it is not. I have tried in the earlier chapters to explain those differences.

Other things that healing is not

- It is not a substitute for veterinary advice or care.
- It is not going to reverse severe degeneration or damage to organs or tissue – all living things have a time span for the physical life to end.
- Nor is healing something that may win more cups or medals for your horse. Improvements to the feeling of general wellbeing may well result in increased success but it should not be the primary reason for healing.

How to give distant healing

There may be a reason why you can't give hands-on healing to your horse. It may be newly acquired and too nervous to approach, or it may be away from home for some reason – to be schooled, or in a veterinary hospital. You may also wish to send healing to a horse you are no longer in contact with but who means a lot to you, or indeed any horse you are concerned about. Healing can be given very effectively from a distance as there is no point at which energy fields emitted from living things actually cease and it is this energy that you can link with and channel healing to. When you concentrate on a particular horse you link with that individual energy field – when you think of horses in general the healing source links with any horse in need.

To give distant healing you need to sit quietly somewhere and focus your thoughts on the horse. If you are not used to meditating then you should find it particularly useful to follow the meditation guidelines detailed in this book as they will help your mind to clear (see page 130). Once you are focused in your mind you can make up your own personal healing prayer of love and comfort – you then quite simply say that you wish for these thoughts to travel to the horse. You may want to say this out loud or in your mind, everyone has their own way of working with distant healing. This healing energy will be received by the horse and it can be very powerful in its benefits. It is something that I do nearly every day and, if possible, I like to have a photo or snippet of mane/tail to help me concentrate on that particular horse. On some occasions people have been with their horse at the same time that I have sent out distant healing and have noted signs that the horse was responding to feeling the healing energy.

With practice, sending out distant healing can become almost second nature and you should find that it becomes very easy to slip into the clear frame of mind needed for sending out some healing thoughts. An important thing to remember is that only a minute or two is needed – it is our intent that is the key.

When we have a spare moment it can be put to good use to help horses everywhere. With distant healing we can send spiritual help to all the thousands of suffering horses in this world even if we do not know who they are or where they are. While sending out thoughts we just need to think something like, 'I wish that the healing energy should go to every horse in need,' and this deep love and compassion will reach them, offering some peace. So spare a minute or two as often as you can (and it can be sitting in a traffic jam or walking in the woods, for example) to send out some healing to help horses everywhere.

Leading a healing life

To be as effective as possible as a healer a person needs to live a healing life. We've all made mistakes, but we do the best in life at a given time based on the information we have and our level of understanding. When we understand more and know a better way, and then do not make changes, is when we fail our horse. That is not to say we won't make more mistakes, we will, because life is a continual learning curve and we evolve as time goes on. But we can say, 'Today is the first day of the rest of my life,' and vow to create a better world for the horse. By doing so in the long run it will be a better world for us too.

Look at the stress in your life and where changes need to be made. Are there people or situations around you that you know aren't good for you? As healers we need to look at every aspect of our lives and where changes need to be made – which situations raise energy levels rather than deplete them. Are there any health issues that need resolving? We need to look after ourselves if we are going to help others, and that includes horses. For optimum healing, diet is important for it is true that we are what we eat.

We need to bear in mind that energy trauma exists in all tissues down to cellular level and the body takes in negative energy from food chain animals kept in bad factory conditions. For healers it is better not to absorb such distressing junk energy.

Earlier in this book we saw how much focus and concentration is required by the healer and how our own energy field is involved in the healing process. To be an efficient healer, and for the work not to deplete or tire us, we need to take good care of our health on all levels. We also need honesty and good intent in our minds and compassion in our hearts. I've found, as many other healers have too, that once on a pathway of giving healing, life begins to take on more meaning and becomes more fulfilling. That doesn't mean to say life won't have its ups and downs, but it will start to have an added dimension. It is just the beginning of something more special.

Simple meditation techniques to aid healing

To strengthen healing potential, regular meditation is necessary to enable the healer to get in touch with the inner self. The more we know our selves and the deeper we can go within, the stronger the healing will become. It will also create inner strength and peace and life should feel enriched. Many people are put off by the idea but it is quite easy to meditate and can improve health as well. Finding the time is important – initially, just 15 minutes of undisturbed time is all that it takes and ideally every day. But if that's not possible then two or three times a week. As you progress and your meditation improves then weekly is fine and ideally extend this special inner healing time to half an hour. See the box overleaf for some advice for enhancing your periods of meditation.

Meditation is a living prayer. You are now beginning to contact your soul and from where your healing will come. As you progress you may see lights or colours. You are then beginning to see energy and healing sources. Keep practising. Your horse needs you to be a healer, and the more you meditate, the more effective you should find that your healing becomes.

'When we experience pure silence in the mind, the body becomes silent also. And in that field of silence healing is much more efficient.'
Deepak Chopra

Useful guidelines for meditation

- Sit quietly somewhere in a comfortable chair. Make sure you are neither too warm nor too cold.
- Switch off the phone or be where you can't hear it.
- Choose a time and a place where other people can't disturb you.
- Exclude animals from this meditation time – it's distracting to have the cat start meowing or the dog start barking just when you get relaxed.
- Don't attempt to meditate after a major upset or trauma, wait until you are calmer.
- Close your eyes and breathe normally.
- Listen to your breathing and let your mind follow it. Is it slow or fast, is it deep or shallow, strong or weak? Let your mind flow with your breath and as you focus on your breath allow your mind to clear. If unwanted thoughts come in then focus again on your breathing, listen to it, the sound it makes and the rhythm, and let those thoughts gently drift away.
- After a while your breathing will change, it may speed up or it may slow down. Follow these changes with your mind. You may feel that your breathing has stopped – which it hasn't, of course. This sensation is because you are now beginning to relax.
- As your breathing slows down allow your arms and legs to become heavy. Eventually, with practice, you will feel as though you are floating, with very slow breathing and a drifting mind.
- Listen to the silence within your mind – realise that you are now contacting your deep source of awareness at the purest level. Now that you have silence in your mind the body is silent also. In that silence healing is at its most efficient. This feeling of deep peace is what you are aiming to achieve in the horse when you give healing.

7
Healing for horses and chakras

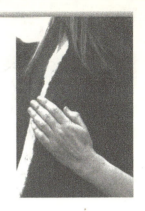

*'All that takes place in nature is permeated
with the mysterious music of the spheres.
In every plant and in every animal
there is really incorporated a tone of the music of the spheres'*

Rudolf Steiner

CHAKRAS ARE THE POINTS OF MAXIMUM ENERGY intake on the body and they have a positive and a negative polarity. Through treating a great number of horses over many years I have been able to establish where there are chakra points on the horse and over these areas I am able to both see and feel the concentration of energy. In Chapter 2 I explained about the layers of vibrating electromagnetic energies in the aura. Each of these is connected to a chakra. If you place your hands an inch or so over these chakra points you should be able to feel under your palms a resistance of energy flowing out from the horse's body.

The word chakra comes from a Sanskrit word meaning 'wheel' because the energy flowing through these points is concentrated with a swirling motion like a wheel, moving both clockwise and anti-clockwise at the same time. However, rather than being circular, the shape of the chakra looks like a flower with several petals – rather like a lotus blossom. A stem of energy from this 'flower' enters the body and attaches to a central core of energy running through the horse's body.

In a healthy horse (and very importantly, it needs to be healthy emotionally as well as physically), the petals of the chakras are open and energy flows freely. Where there is imbalance, energies become blocked. Healing channelled over the chakras of the horse aims to open and clear these energy centres, helping to create physical, mental and emotional

HEALING FOR HORSES

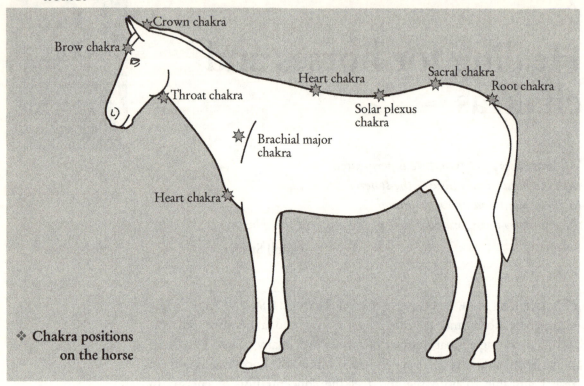

❖ Chakra positions on the horse

harmony for the horse. By treating each chakra you can give the horse a full healing treatment.

How to give the horse healing over the chakras

You need to first prepare yourself by following the meditation techniques for at least a week as outlined in Chapter 6. This will help to focus your mind and clear some of your own energy junk. Then I would recommend first practising on a human as this is much better than working initially on a fidgety horse, and allows you the chance to feel the chakra energy.

Ask a sympathetic friend or relative to sit comfortably in a quiet room and stand behind them with your eyes closed. Allow all thoughts to drift away and imagine you are looking at a golden ball of light like the sun. Then open your eyes and place your hand over the top of the person's head about six inches away. Slowly move your hand closer until you feel your hand pushed up. Some people may feel heat or a prickly sensation, or even a pulse. When you feel one or more of these things move on to the fore-

HEALING FOR HORSES AND CHAKRAS

head, and then over the abdomen. Be patient, these sensations are very subtle and you also need to have an open mind. Allow yourself to work intuitively. Does your hand want to move further back or forward, or to one side? Work slowly and gently, going with the flow as this is what the body needs – keep the treatment short, about 20 minutes total. Now you are ready to go out to give healing to your horse through the chakras.

Where to begin on the horse

You can begin healing at any chakra but I recommend starting at the brachial major chakra, then moving on to either the solar plexus or heart chakras, until you get more experienced at feeling the energy and the changes. Begin by placing your hand very gently over the chakra points about an inch away then gradually lower your hand to touch the horse very softly and gently. Some healers prefer to use their finger tips and if that is how you find you like to work that is fine.

What you may feel

As you work with the healing you should feel the changes as the chakra responds and rebalances. There may be sensations of tingling or heat, or your hand may feel heavy. If your hand is pushed upwards, the healing treatment has been effective over that chakra and you can move on to the next one.

Don't be despondent if you seem to feel very little at first – these are subtle sensations and some people feel them more quickly than others. It takes time to adjust to a new way of feeling and many healers take years to fully develop their skills.

You should find it most rewarding to work with your horse in this way and over a period of time there should be noticeable improvements in your horse's sense of wellbeing. You can give healing this way weekly or for the injured or sick horse daily. Keep the treatments at 20 to 30 minutes initially and then increase to up to an hour if necessary. As with anything, practice makes for a stronger response.

Chakra healing as first aid

Chakra healing can be given as a first aid and I have found this very effective. If your horse is in shock, has just been injured or has suddenly gone down with a health problem place your hand or fingers over the crown, brow or brachial major chakra, if possible, until the vet arrives. Focus with your mind on healing the horse and helping it through this stressful time. When giving first aid healing you may feel an abnormal pulsing sensation under your hand or fingers as the disturbed energy resonates out of rhythm.

Affirmations

I have included some affirmations linked to each chakra. What are affirmations? They are words that help us to focus our minds on a spiritual level – prayers that raise our consciousness. These prayers are aimed at opening up our heart chakra, through which we give healing. Affirmations are words of compassion and love, and they link our mind with our spiritual self, thereby creating an *intent* to help and heal. Through this strengthening and combining of intent and focus the healing energy is linked to the horse on all possible levels.

The affirmations I have included are only suggestions but they have worked well for me. You can use your own words, and you can use affirmations to help your healing in general, not just when working through the chakras. Affirmations can be very simple; for example, just saying 'I love you' to a horse has a very powerful energy pattern. Words of love and good intent will help raise the vibrations around you and your horse, and link you in a spiritual sense to help your healing. The important thing is to really mean what you are saying and to keep the affirmations on a spiritual level.

Colours, planets or elements and the chakras

Chakras are an ancient Indian concept used to explain energy currents in the body and as a map of consciousness. Linking with chakra energy is a common practice in yoga and other forms of meditation. When I was developing as a healer we always started and finished our classes by concentrating on the chakra system and its relevant colours. It is historically accepted that there are seven major chakras situated along the length of the body, and both Eastern and Western traditions acknowledge

HEALING FOR HORSES AND CHAKRAS

that there are many more in addition to these. Each chakra has a colour, planet and part of the body associated with it. The physical link is to the organs that lie in the vicinity of the chakra in question, or whose energy flows through that chakra. The original seven chakras have colours that together make up the colours of the rainbow. However, any colour may be seen or sensed in the chakra as the flow of energy changes and this can give us information about the physical, emotional and spiritual health of the person or animal.

The elements or planets that relate to each chakra vary according to different sources, so I have used the ones with which I have been most familiar over the years. These elements and planets possess qualities and natural energies that are compatible with the pattern of the chakra that they are linked with.

When I discovered the existence of what I've come to call the brachial major chakra in horses and other animals, I knew it would be linked to a particular colour, planet and part of the body. Because of its anatomical position, it was easy to tell what part of the body it was linked to, but determining the planet and colour was – I knew – going to be hard! I meditated, asking for the answer to be shown to me. After a day or two I remembered that one of my clients, Pamela, was a highly qualified astrologer, so I called her for advice. I explained that I knew that the brachial major chakra was a very powerful centre of energy and through it you could treat the whole body, yet it was also linked to every other chakra. It was also an area where I could get a strong release of emotional energy. 'What planet could this describe?' I asked.

Immediately, Pamela answered, 'Pluto,' explaining that Pluto exerts a powerful influence and acts as a catalyst and intensifier on the planets that it aspects. It is the planet of transformation. This transformation can be symbolic, or the actual end of an episode or physical life. (It was over this chakra that I felt the life force, or soul, leave a cat recently when he died.) After a Pluto transit something always changes; nothing is ever the same. So that would explain this chakra's very spiritual role in releasing and re-balancing the emotions, and its link to the other chakras. I asked Pamela what colour would be associated with this planet and she said black, because it is associated with darkness into light, coming back to the transformation link again.

Now I had a problem with black, as it seemed so severe and not like the bright colours of the other chakras. I mulled over it and a week later the confirmation came. I was treating Ygrec, a black Labrador dog, who has regular healing for his arthritis. When I treat him, I am always joined by six-year-old twins Alexander and Victoria. Alexander has a slight physical disability and I link him with the healing I give Ygrec to help him in his life too. Young children can get very bored so I turn the healing sessions into a game. On this occasion I decided to get the children to concentrate on what colours they could see during the healing. Victoria calls the tingling from the healing energy 'fairy dust' – a very apt description – so I laid my hands on Ygrec and the twins put their hands on his head and waited for the 'fairy dust' to appear. I asked them to tell me what colours they could see over the various chakras and was amazed at their accuracy in getting each one correct. I wondered what they would sense over the brachial major chakra and, holding my hand over it, asked them to look underneath and tell me what colour was there. Very solemnly Victoria studied the area and, looking at me, said, 'Black.' Alexander said he could see black too. I realised then that through the innocence and openness of these special children I had received my answer as to the colour associated with the brachial major chakra. And of course the sum total of all colours is black too, so that made sense as it links all the other chakras.

The brachial major chakra

This is a chakra that I discovered early on when starting to give healing to horses. At first I didn't realise that it was a chakra area, but I was always drawn back to this point where I found I could access the horse's whole energy field very quickly. I have named this the brachial major chakra because anatomically it accesses the brachial plexus of nerves, an important network innervating the head, neck, chest and forelimbs. Through this chakra I have found that I can access all the other chakras, which is useful when treating a very nervous horse that can't be touched anywhere else. This chakra seems to relate to the horse's relationship with mankind so is a very important area through which to channel healing. The brachial major chakra lies at each side of the horse's neck, in the dip just above the shoulder. In the very sensitive or worried horse I may give healing just by contact with this area.

HEALING FOR HORSES AND CHAKRAS

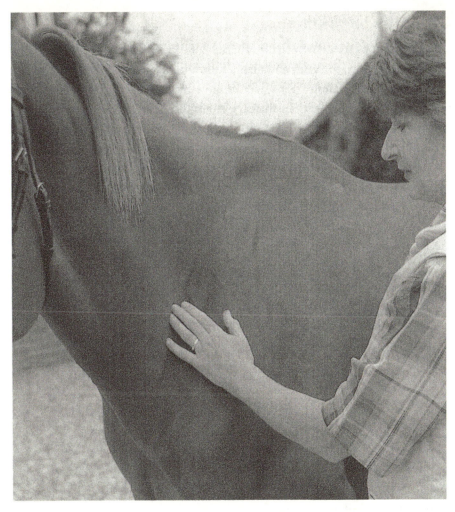

The position of the brachial major chakra.

The brachial major chakra

Location: each side of the horse's neck in the dip just above the shoulder
Key words relating to the horse: relationship to mankind, instinct, healing, unity, awareness, magnetism, energy intensifies
Colour: black
Planet: Pluto
Element: the universe
Sense: the instincts
Physical connection to the horse: head, neck, chest, forelimbs
Gemstone: carnelian, tiger's eye, snowflake, obsidian
Affirmation to the horse: 'We are united as children of the universe. May the energy embrace us and transform so that we emerge stronger in spirit.'

HEALING FOR HORSES

The crown chakra

At the point of the crown chakra there is a reflection of the life force or soul of the horse into the aura and also a link with a divine intelligence, so this is an important chakra over which to give healing. This chakra lies on top of the horse's head between the ears. Many horses are head shy and worry about this area being touched, even for healing, and that means there could possibly be a structural problem, so ask your vet to check and possibly refer to a physiotherapist, chiropractor or osteopath. You can also access this energy area in the horse by holding your hand over the brow chakra as well, which I find most horses do not object to.

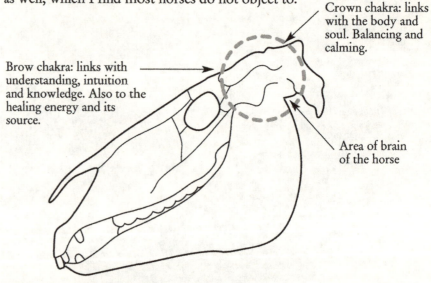

Chakras on the head of the horse

Brow chakra: links with understanding, intuition and knowledge. Also to the healing energy and its source.

Crown chakra: links with the body and soul. Balancing and calming.

Area of brain of the horse

The crown chakra

Location: top of the head between the ears

Key words relating to the horse: calmness, soul, spirit, peace, balance, release, wisdom

Colour: violet

Planet: Uranus

Element: gold

Sense: thought

Physical connection to the horse: centre of the brain (pituitary – master gland), central nervous system, cranio-sacral system, spine, skin and hair

Gemstone: amethyst, diamond, white tourmaline, snowy quartz, celestite

Affirmation to the horse: 'I wish you complete peace and harmony. May you be at ease with the world and at one with the universe.'

HEALING FOR HORSES
AND CHAKRAS

The brow chakra

I use this chakra to bless the horse and help it to feel the love from the universal source of healing, which I call God. When energies flow freely here it allows the horse a chance to understand the purpose of everything in its life. This chakra will be closed in stressed and depressed horses. The brow chakra is situated in the centre of the forehead above the eyes.

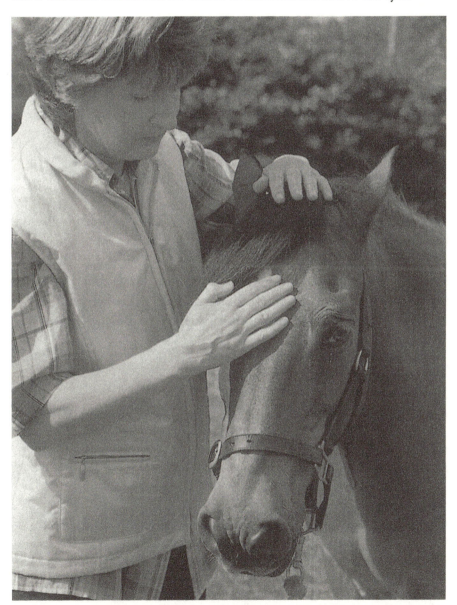

Hands over the brow and crown chakras, giving healing to a 35-year-old pony to help with arthritis.

The brow chakra

Location: across the forehead above the eyes
Key words relating to the horse: understanding, insight, sense of wholeness, link to the universe, completeness, imagination, intuition, knowledge
Colour: indigo or purple
Planet: Jupiter
Element: silver
Sense: intuition
Physical connection to the horse: centre of the brain (pineal – the gland that controls body rhythms including sleeping and waking. Daylight important for the function of pineal), higher mental self.
Gemstone: amethyst, pearl, blue flourite, white flourite
Affirmation to the horse: 'May you be blessed with understanding of your life. I promise that I will do my best for you.'

The throat chakra

The throat chakra can be easily blocked as the horse struggles to communicate with the people in its life. It is an area that needs healing in horses who are or have been denied adequate contact with other horses as they cannot express themselves naturally. The throat chakra is found across the throat, but never hold, grip or pinch; hold your hand slightly below this area to give the healing. Healing here helps to prevent negative energy from affecting the horse on a physical as well as mental/emotional level.

The throat chakra

Location: just under lower jaw across the throat
Key words relating to the horse: communication, expression, release, creativity, healing
Colour: blue
Planet: Mercury
Element: the heavens
Sense: hearing
Physical connection to the horse: ears, nose, mouth, teeth, thyroid area, throat
Gemstone: turquoise, sapphire, aquamarine, lapis lazuli
Affirmation to the horse: 'I ask that my responsibility is clear enough to allow me to hear your communication. You can let me know how you feel and I will heal you.'

HEALING FOR HORSES AND CHAKRAS

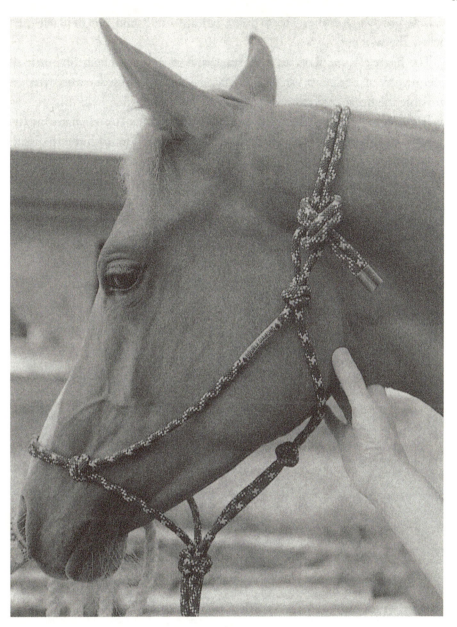

The throat chakra. Keep the fingers slightly away from the horse. Never apply pressure to, or hold, this area.

The heart chakra

This is a very important area as the healer's own heart chakra is always open when giving healing, because it is the energy centre through which we give and receive love. I have found that the heart chakra is best accessed by placing the hand on the centre of the horse's chest, in the middle of the muscle groove. Another access point can also be found on the back just below the withers.

The heart chakra plays an important role in the movement of spiritual energies from healer to horse. For changes in life to be as stress free as possible the heart chakra needs to be open, so give healing over this area as well as over the solar plexus chakra before and after any changes in the horse's life or routine. It is one to treat after weaning in both the foal and

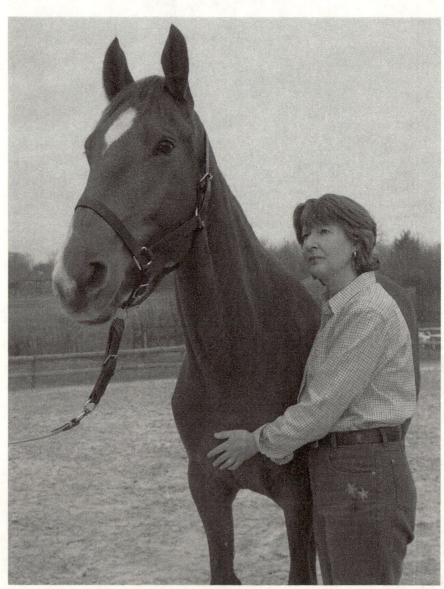

Giving healing through the heart chakra. This is where I have found it best to access this chakra.

the mare, before you introduce new equines, after loss of the horse's friend or change of home and definitely for giving to a new horse in your life.

It is a very important point on the horse to give healing and any healing session should include this area. Through this chakra the horse can let go of energy disturbance and obstruction, which in the human would have resulted in crying. Through this chakra I have frequently been able to release emotional blockages in the horse. On those occasions people watching have often become tearful as they feel the sadness leave the horse. Pain, shock, hospitalisation, loneliness, stress, over-stabling, mental and physical abuse, etc., all shut down the energy flow through this chakra.

The heart chakra

Location: centre of the chest area and just below the withers
Key words relating to the horse: love, feeling, forgiveness, tenderness, emotion, sharing, balance (body, mind, spirit)
Colour: green
Planet: Venus
Element: air
Sense: touch, feeling
Physical connection to the horse: heart, lungs, thymus (a gland of the lymphatic system, plays a vital role in the immune system)
Gemstone: emerald, azurite, jade, tourmaline
Affirmation to the horse: 'I love you. Feel my love and let it warm and protect you always.'

The solar plexus chakra

This is another chakra affected by the emotional state and when giving healing through the solar plexus chakra I have been able to facilitate many horses' energy releases, which have resulted in behavioural improvements and increased wellbeing. Energy blockage around this area affects the digestive organs and upsets in these organs also close down the solar plexus chakra. Often when healing in this area there are tummy rumbling noises or releases of wind as the energy begins to clear. It is an important chakra to treat after a competition as adrenaline in the system and the 'flight and fight' syndrome (which gives us a feeling of butterflies in the tummy) can block this chakra. I find that the solar plexus chakra is situated in the centre of the back, midway between the heart and sacral chakras.

HEALING FOR HORSES

The solar plexus chakra

Location: in the centre of the back
Key words relating to the horse: release of emotions, reason, freedom of spirit, survival, will power, sense of purpose, energy
Colour: yellow
Planet: Mars
Element: fire
Sense: sight
Physical connection to the horse: whole body, digestive system, stomach, liver
Gemstone: amber, citrine, topaz, rose quartz, moonstone, garnet, alexandrite
Affirmation to the horse: 'I set your spirit free and release your tears to the universe. I offer you calmness and strength.'

The sacral chakra

I have found that a great deal of unbalanced emotional and mental energy can be released through giving healing to this chakra. It is a centre that has a role in security and nurturing and anatomically is at the end of the cranio-sacral system so is affected by these rhythms of the body and vice versa. Any injury/shock to the spine or head injury will also shut down this chakra. This chakra lies in the centre of the sacral (hip) region of the spine.

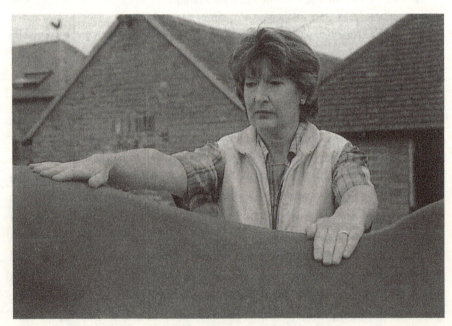

Giving healing through the heart chakra (left hand) and sacral chakra (right hand).

The sacral chakra

Location: across the top of the pelvis (hips)
Key words relating to the horse: security, release, creativity, empowerment, sense of others, sense of sexuality, emotions, desire
Colour: orange
Planet: Moon
Element: water
Sense: taste
Physical connection to the horse: lymphatic system, kidneys, adrenal glands, reproductive system
Gemstone: amber, citrine, topaz, moonstone, jasper, ruby
Affirmation to the horse: 'We are joined as one in the universal energy. I release your body from negative energy.'

The root chakra

This is the seventh chakra and it is where we give healing to ground the horse. It also helps the confusion we have created in the horse's life regarding responses to instincts and natural elements. Any physical problems in the horse, including musculo-skeletal damage, will affect this chakra. I give healing through this chakra by placing my hand at the end of the back where the tail starts.

The root chakra

Location: at the bottom of the back where the tail starts
Key words relating to the horse: grounding, stability, acceptance, self-preservation, physical strength
Colour: red
Planet: Saturn
Element: earth
Sense: smell
Physical connection to the horse: legs, feet, intestines
Gemstone: bloodstone, agate, tiger's eye, garnet, alexandrite, onyx, smoky quartz, ruby
Affirmation to the horse: 'May your life force be re-charged and strengthened. Accept this healing.'

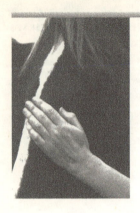

8
Crystals and gemstones for healing

'Let us be crystal clear about our good intentions for our horses'
                                        Margrit Coates

NATURAL CRYSTALS and gemstones have an energy of their own which can be useful in healing for horses and we can make use of these energies for certain conditions. It is important to realise that in the tissue of mammals, including horses, there are living crystals with vibratory properties compatible with crystal stones. Liquid crystal molecules form cell membranes, nerve sheaths, connective tissue, fasciae, collagen and fibrous components. When we use crystal stones they have resonant interactions with the liquid crystals within the tissues of the horse and so can enhance the therapeutic effects. As with all forms of healing it is absolutely vital that the healer's intent is to help for totally unselfish reasons. This applies to the use of crystals and gemstones – they must be used for the benefit of the horse holistically to have any real meaning. Tune in to the higher power when holding them over the horse and let the healing energies flow. I recommend using just one or two stones per healing session for maximum effect. If any of the stones relate to health problems you have yourself then you can use them to give yourself healing the day before you treat a horse, so that you are better balanced yourself.

I do not advise using crystals as a treatment by itself but to incorporate these stones as an added extra to be used with your hands-on healing. This is because nothing can beat the simplicity and power of hands-on healing, which treats on all levels within the horse. The use of crystals can subtly enhance some of the natural energies.

On pages 148–9, I have listed the stones that I have found most useful when healing with horses.

CRYSTALS AND
GEMSTONES FOR HEALING

Remember the golden rule

If you are concerned about the health or wellbeing of your horse consult your vet. Don't try other things first and lose valuable time when the horse may need veterinary help.

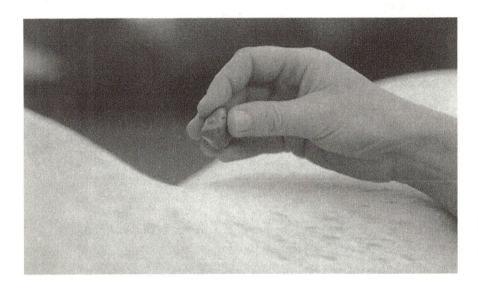

The use of crystals or gemstones can enhance the subtle energies during hands-on healing sessions.

How to use the stones

You can carry a small one in your pocket when you are riding or working with the horse or wear one round your neck. I have found the best ones to wear are amethyst, rose quartz and amber. Amethyst is the stone with the strongest overall healing energy and is good to use for chakra healing with convalescing horses or depleted horses. It is also a good stone to wear for the owner who is run down or in low spirits. If there is a shelf or ledge in the stable I have often placed a stone or two securely on it. Also when you are giving healing over the chakras you can hold a small stone in your hand to enhance the benefits.

Cleanse all stones first by leaving them under a running cold tap for ten minutes and then leave in natural daylight to dry – it is even better if you can leave them under a full moon for a night. Every fortnight you need to re-cleanse the stones to wash out negative energy.

Healing qualities of stones for use with horses

- **Agate**: for strength of purpose and joie de vivre. Useful for depressed and sad horses, barren mares, brood mares and stud stallions.
- **Alexandrite**: helps wounds and injuries to heal and tissues to regenerate. Use for injuries and also for bereavement, loss of companions, life's changes, etc.
- **Amber**: my favourite as it is native to my ancestors' homeland in Prussia. A powerful stone (actually it's a resin), it is good for energising, balancing and healing. Use for depressed or tense horses and those with emotional problems. Good for mares in season and stallions as it links with the reproductive organs.
- **Amethyst**: promotes healing and links with the higher consciousness. It is a stone for protection as it helps disperse negative energy.
- **Aquamarine**: fears and phobias. Use for healing with nervous horses.
- **Azurite**: linked to the air. Use for COPD, allergies, breathing problems and sinusitis.
- **Bloodstone**: cleansing and purifying. Use for liver problems and post-viral syndrome. Also good for competition horses.
- **Blue flourite**: for protection. Use for shielding your horse from negative energy.
- **Carnelian**: strengthens the horse's link to natural spiritual elements. Useful for depressed horses and those in shock. Use over the brachial major chakra.
- **Celestite**: promotes vitality. A balancing stone, use it over the crown chakra.
- **Citrine**: for clarity, for treating the solar plexus. Also use over the sacral area for digestive problems and colicky horses.
- **Diamond**: for perfection. Use to balance the horse.
- **Emerald**: for wisdom, loyalty and trust. Use if you need to build up a bond with the horse.
- **Garnet**: see alexandrite.
- **Jade**: linked to the life force, it helps the heart energy and general vitality.
- **Jasper**: for empowerment. Use for balancing the whole body over the sacral chakra.

CRYSTALS AND GEMSTONES FOR HEALING

- **Lapis lazuli**: for expression, it is linked to hearing as well. Useful for lack of confidence or nervous horses.
- **Moonstone**: for inner feelings. A stone to use to help develop friendship with the horse.
- **Onyx**: for stamina. Use with post-viral conditions, low immune system, poor doers.
- **Pearl**: aids serenity and purification of thought. It is one to use for blessing your horse with peace.
- **Rose quartz**: the universal healing and clearing stone. Can be used over any chakra for bringing peace and tranquillity to the horse and for balancing. It is especially good for healing problems relating to geopathic conditions (see Chapter 3).
- **Ruby**: revitalises. Use after a difficult foaling, for both foal and mare.
- **Sapphire**: for communication at all levels. Use over the throat chakra.
- **Smoky quartz**: for calmness and grounding. It is helpful for panic and shock so use for highly strung equines and in first aid.
- **Snow flake obsidian**: to strengthen in times of change. It is a stone that relates to the cycle of life and death (and rebirth). A good stone to use for the very sick horse, also those with low immune systems.
- **Snowy quartz**: for loneliness or resentment. For troubled equines or those kept away from other horses. Also during box rest for injury or illness.
- **Tiger's eye**: creativity. Use for nervous and working horses, especially before a show or competition.
- **Topaz**: a fertility stone. Use with barren mares, or mares to be mated.
- **Tourmaline**: aids compassion and tolerance. Helpful for the horse after a loss, bereavement or other trauma.
- **Turquoise**: relates to mind-body communication. It is another stone to use to help strengthen your bond with the horse.
- **White flourite**: to strengthen the spirit of the horse. Use for any equine with history of bad treatment.
- **White tourmaline**: for spiritual enlightenment. Use to help promote a sense of wellbeing at the deepest level.

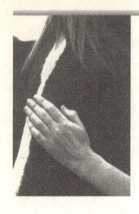

9
Other natural therapies

*'Let me look back and to my conscience say
because of some kind act to beast or man
the world is better that I lived today'*

Anon

BECAUSE OF THE COMPLEXITY of a horse's problems it is essential that a vet makes the initial diagnosis. Subsequently that vet is able to call upon other members of the therapeutic team, including the farrier, saddler, dentist, osteopath, physiotherapist, chiropractor, trainer, healer and not least the rider. Through good interdisciplinary communication the sum will be greater then the individual parts.

Depending on the condition, healing can sometimes set up a process of repair and recovery that may stimulate enough improvements to be effective without involvement from other therapies in the 'holistic team' – all of which operate on individual levels to promote better health and improved wellbeing. However, the team approach is very beneficial and, in many cases, essential. Other therapies may treat individual symptoms or work to influence changes on all levels. All will affect the energy field of the horse in some way.

It is always helpful to use healing to work alongside any other treatments that the horse may be having as pain and discomfort are very stressful, depressing and debilitating. Sometimes tension can aggravate pain and discomfort and healing can help the horse to relax and let go of emotional and other energy blockages. Also if the horse has disturbed mental or emotional energy or is harbouring anger, resentment, grief or fear, then these feelings may prevent other therapies from working as best they can. Every part of the horse's body works from the sum total of the whole so if one area is disturbed it will have a knock-on effect somewhere else.

There are many therapies with which healing works very well and that I have been fortunate to have experience of, alongside those listed overleaf.

OTHER NATURAL THERAPIES

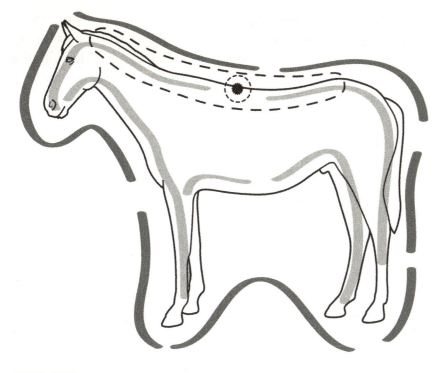

The effect of therapies that use energy on the horse's body, using back pain as an example.

▬▬▬ Hands-on healing treats the whole horse on an emotional, mental and physical level to aim for homeostasis. When one part of the energy field is blocked it will affect the whole.

▬▬▬ Homeopathic and herbal remedies work at all levels in a holistic way as well as being able to target specific areas.

– – – – Acupuncture needles are inserted into channels or meridians specific to the source of pain, helping reduce inflammation and give pain relief.

- - - - - - Physiotherapy machines such as laser and ultrasound concentrate energy around the site of application to stimulate tissue repair.

Healing works in the energy field of the horse affecting all the different aspects at once, to aim for establishing homeostasis, or balance. The way I look at it is that this then gives a blank piece of paper for the other treatments to work on. So, in effect, these therapies are not working against unbalanced energy but with balanced energy. This means that the treatments may be more effective, and can work at the deepest level.

Occasionally, therapies produce a 'healing crisis', which means that the condition can temporarily get worse before it gets better, as things are aggravated. This is not the case, however, with healing by the laying on of hands. In my experience the horse may be quieter for a while after healing or even more energised, but the response should be positive as things are not disturbed but balanced during this treatment. Healing aims to give the horse balanced energy and other therapies can then make good use of that energy.

All the therapies listed below may only be carried out with permission from a veterinary surgeon to safeguard your horse and to ensure that only qualified people are used.

Acupuncture

This is an ancient form of medicine going back nearly 3000 years, which originated in China. In humans it is the most popular alternative therapy, used by millions of people a year, and as a result more and more vets are training in and offering acupuncture for horses. Very fine needles are used on specific points and nervous or anxious horses may need to be sedated first. When the needle reaches the acupuncture point there is often a sensation like a dull ache and some horses may find this uncomfortable without sedation. I've watched many horses receiving acupuncture and usually they find it very relaxing. In the horses that I've treated with healing that were also having acupuncture, I have usually given the healing on a different day. However, in some acute cases I've given healing (to help stimulate the energy lines) just before the vet applied acupuncture to try and help the efficacy of the treatment. Healing usually has a sedating effect anyway so can be beneficial in these cases as well.

Acupuncture works holistically in the energy field of the horse, as does healing. The classical Chinese explanation is that channels of energy run in regular patterns through the body and over the surface. These channels are called meridians and during a healing session I may work over these lines to stimulate them as well as working generally in the energy field. Scientific research done on acupuncture meridians shows that they are where electricity flows in a low resistance and when I'm healing I can often feel with my hands the electrical changes over these areas. Meridian channels extend right through to the heart of every cell in the body and healers can make use of these channels in the horse. During an acupuncture treatment needles stimulate points along the meridians, which triggers the release of chemicals and hormones, influencing the horse's internal regulating system. Healing is compatible with acupuncture as both are balancing therapies, and both work with the bio-electrical movement of the body to promote a natural return to health.

OTHER NATURAL THERAPIES

In the UK only a veterinary surgeon may administer acupuncture to a horse; it is against the Veterinary Act for anyone else to do so.

Homeopathy

Like acupuncture, homeopathy treats the whole body. Homeopaths and healers recognise subtle energy in the living body which homeopaths call the 'vital force', the force running through the body responsible for its healthy function and defence against disease. In homeopathy, as in healing, this concept is fundamental to understanding how the treatment works.

A homeopathic vet will take a full consultation case history to establish what type the horse is so that a constitutional remedy can be prescribed. Specific remedies and herbs for individual problems can also be offered and these will be prescribed in different potencies depending on the vet's diagnosis. Homeopaths further believe in 'miasms', the chronic effect of an underlying disease, which has been present in previous generations. Healers may refer to this as karma. Homeopathy relies on the energy of the individual remedy to work with the vital force of the horse whereas healers work in general terms within the energy field.

By working alongside homeopathic vets, I have found that homeopathic remedies can be more effective in some cases when used with sessions of healing as the healing calms and clears away energy blockages so that the remedies can go in deeper. For example, with this combination we've had particular success with epilepsy, post-viral syndrome, infections, tumours, shock and injury and behavioural problems. Homeopathy is a very potent form of medicine and has none of the adverse side effects associated with orthodox drugs – therefore healing and homeopathy make a very powerful combination.

As with acupuncture, only a veterinary surgeon may prescribe homeopathic remedies or herbs for a horse.

Physiotherapy

Equine physiotherapists will be chartered physiotherapists, which means that they have undergone extensive full-time training to degree level and worked with humans before taking a further post-graduate course in animal physiotherapy. Equine physiotherapists specialise in treating the musculo-skeletal system of the horse. Examples of horses needing physiotherapy include those with mobility or schooling problems, those suffering from age-related stiffness, competition horses and, of course, any horse who has had an accident. Regular physiotherapy is also invaluable in helping prevent injury in horses as it keeps the musculo-skeletal system functioning at the best possible level. Many of today's equine physiotherapists are also extending their knowledge into the field of energy medicine and may use subtle techniques to aid recovery in the horse – for example, cranio-sacral therapy or the use of laser and electrotherapy stimulation. Physiotherapy works mechanically within the energy field running through the muscles, ligaments, tendons and bones of the horse and therefore healing can prepare or help to maintain strong energy in these areas, stimulating soft tissue repair.

At Holistic Pets we have several equine physiotherapists in the practice and we have found that healing can help their work in many ways. It can help speed up the repair of soft tissue injury and stimulate the immune system where inflammation is present. Where the horse has injured its back, healing is useful to rebalance the energy that flows through the centre of the spine. Sometimes the physiotherapists have asked me to give healing to a horse because they felt that some emotional blockage was preventing their treatment from being fully effective as the tissues were holding on to their memories of trauma. Healing in these cases releases the negative emotional energy allowing the physiotherapist to go in at a deeper level and make the desired adjustments. Physiotherapy and healing can be a very effective combination for the older arthritic horse helping to give improved mobility and natural pain relief, thereby improving the sense of wellbeing.

I give healing treatments to the horse either on a different day to physiotherapy or if on the same day, after a physiotherapist has treated first. In the early days I sometimes gave healing to a horse before the physiotherapist treated it thinking it would calm the horse and get a good energy flow. However the physiotherapists found that when they went to do the hands-on assessment around the horse's body there was not enough energy tension for them to be able to work with; they couldn't in effect feel anything – the horse's system was too relaxed.

Massage

Members of the Equine Sports Massage Association are qualified equine sports massage therapists who have first undertaken training to treat humans and then taken a post-graduate course to treat horses. Equine sports massage is the application of professional massage techniques to the horse to improve circulation and muscle tone, prevent or relieve adhesions and encourage freedom of movement. By using their hands the therapists have constant feedback from the tissues they are massaging so each session will be varied according to the needs of the horse.

Used before exertion sports, massage ensures that the muscles are in the best condition to perform. After exertion, massage aids the removal of toxic by-products of exercise so minimising stiffness and fatigue, and used after injury, massage stimulates the circulation to aid repair of tissue. Regular massage as part of a training programme helps to minimise the risk of injury as well as enhancing performance by enabling the horse to use muscles more economically and smoothly. As a qualified massage therapist myself I really appreciate the benefits that regular treatments can give to relax and reduce stress levels.

Osteopathy

Osteopathy is a discipline involving the diagnosis of structural problems in humans and animals. Attention is generally, though by no means always exclusively, directed to the spine. In the UK, the osteopath's training over four years leads to a BSc degree and introduction to the application of osteopathy to animals is studied at post-graduate level.

Horses suffer injuries to the neck, back and pelvis for many reasons, among which feature accidents and inappropriate use. Once traumatised, the spinal joint complex becomes stiff and functions poorly – this may be immediately obvious, but in many cases the changes are subtle. An example of a horse with stiff spinal joints is the competition horse who, although not lame, under-achieves or may move better to one side or the other. Over time these subtle changes and poor function of spinal joints increase the effort in other areas of the spine. In other words, the spine compensates but it can only do this up to a certain point – once passed, the compensation breaks down and the horse suddenly shows signs of being unable to perform appropriately. Back problems can also be secondary to foot or limb trouble. A vet must always make the initial diagnosis before referral to an equine osteopath. I am personally very interested in osteopathy and its benefits and it is a treatment I have myself on a regular basis.

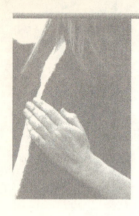

10
Using a healer for your horse

*'You are not alone
the centuries fight for you
eternity is your ally –
You are in the keeping of the one
who holds you with love
that will not let you go'*

Joseph R. Sizoo

A VERY IMPORTANT THING to remember is that a healer does not diagnose and hands-on healing is not a substitute for veterinary advice – a vet should always be consulted first for any problems. Registered healers operate within a strict code of conduct which states that they should not visit a horse without making prior enquiry that it has been examined by and is under the care of a veterinary surgeon. In the UK, the Royal College of Veterinary Surgeons publishes a guide with information about the use of faith healing and this information can be found in paragraph 18 of part 2F. In the USA, each state has its own laws regarding the use of complementary therapies, which a vet can advise on. Where possible I give demonstrations of healing to vets so that they can experience for themselves what happens during a treatment.

The vet must be the first port of call with any concerns over your horse's health, behaviour or wellbeing. As well as not being qualified to make a diagnosis, healers may not prescribe medication – that is the prerogative of a veterinary surgeon. There are many reasons why the horse may appear unwell or change its behaviour and your vet can check these.

Registered healers

You may wish to call in the services of a professional healer, and as with using any practitioner of complementary therapies, it is important that you

USING A HEALER FOR YOUR HORSE

have a rapport and a trust with the therapist. Healers come in all shapes and sizes as they are human beings. They will have their own personalities and it is best to choose one who you feel at ease with, otherwise when that person comes to treat your horse you will feel tense and the horse will pick up on that. Each healer will have their own way of working, which they find is best for them, normally laying the hands on the horse. However, around the horse is a force field that consists of subtle energies and sometimes a healer may need to step back to work on one of these subtle fields, which lie a little way out from the body. Some healers use their fingertips and others the palm of the hand and mostly I use a combination of these methods. Most healers today adopt a non-denominational approach to their work recognising that everyone has their own beliefs to follow – and the horse has no concept of faiths, religions or doctrines anyway.

I suggest telephoning the healer first, and don't be afraid to ask questions about how they work and their experience. For healing with horses I believe it is absolutely essential that the healer has some experience and understanding of horses. Horses are unpredictable animals and I'd be very rich indeed if I had a pound for every time someone said to me, 'It's never done that before.' It's always a potentially dangerous situation giving healing to a horse so for everyone's safety it is better that your healer has an awareness of the nature of horses and is confident in their presence.

Professional healers will make a charge for giving healing to your horse and this is to cover their time and travelling expenses. It doesn't stop there either. As well as the actual time spent with the horse there are several more hours spent attending to paperwork, phone calls, faxes, etc. associated with each visit. Registered healers have also spent a great deal of time and money undergoing training and taking courses to develop their abilities to a high level. They also have registration fees and public liability insurance to pay for. Often they are practitioners of other therapies or disciplines and are very busy people. Healers may offer concessions – I give healing treatments voluntarily to horses that belong to rescue organisations or charities.

A healer who belongs to a recognised association works to a strict code of conduct and this is some safeguard as you are inviting a stranger to your home or yard. Calling in a healer from an association means that someone has checked out this person and that they have undergone a specified length of time developing their potential as a healer. They will understand how to work with healing energies and be proficient in harnessing those energies. Registered healers are also aware of the Veterinary Act and will work within guidelines relating to this. As required by my healer membership I always fill in a client record sheet with details of the horse and its history. If you are interested in having healing for your horse then you should mention this to your vet – most have an open mind and would be interested in benefits that you notice.

It is a good idea to have a healing treatment yourself so that you can experience what it feels like, and we can all do with regular rebalancing in the very stressful world which we live in today. I have a healing treatment monthly and certainly feel the benefit from a session; it's like having a week's holiday in an hour.

How many healing treatments will the healer give?

This will depend on the condition being treated, the response from the horse and the way the healer is able to channel the energy. For example, chronic conditions will generally need more sessions than acute ones. I find that if the horse's problem is emotionally based then one to three treatments are usually enough. I often have people ask me to come and see a healthy horse for no reason other than they would like it to have healing and in this case one treatment is usually enough to rebalance the horse. It is very beneficial for seemingly healthy horses to have a healing session as healing can be used as a preventative measure. The idea is that by keeping the physical and emotional energies balanced the horse will have a stronger immune system, be less accident prone and any injuries will repair more quickly. I have given healing to competition horses before a major race or event and owners have reported an increase in vitality and energy, so that is also a time to consider using healing.

Both before and after any major changes to the horse's life is a good time to call a healer. It helps the horse to deal with the disturbed emotional energy, which in the long term can lead to physical or behavioural problems. We can talk about our problems and have a good cry, which the horse cannot do, and healing releases all that energy and stops it from getting pent up. Certainly if your horse loses a friend I would always recommend healing for helping it to get over the loss.

For chronic conditions, such as tumours, post-viral syndrome, arthritis, infections and injuries, I would visit on a regular basis until the situation improved, then cut down to a maintenance visit every few weeks until the horse was better. Obviously this is the way that I work and every healer is different.

For the terminally ill horse healing is invaluable and offers peace in the last stages of life's journey. When the owner knows that a horse is very sick and time is short it is a good idea to call a healer. I would treat as soon as possible, then, depending on how much time was left, weekly or more often until the end. Healing can be given in this way on the last day just before the vet makes the final visit. It offers the horse a feeling of inner tranquillity and natural pain relief and this can help the owners too during this very sad and traumatic time.

Finally, healers will not make promises about a cure or recovery. It has been shown that healing can make a contribution to recovery but each case is individual and no predictions as to a result can ever be made. Sometimes a return to a previous level of health is not possible but healing aims to strengthen the process to the best possible level. A rebalancing of energy can allow the animal's own healing resources to activate and strengthen resulting in a return to homeostasis. Basically you can use a healer for any condition that your horse has a problem with, and sometimes I'm asked to give healing treatment because all else has failed.

Every healer has his or her own way of working, a style and technique that they will have developed with experience that works best for them. However, the basics will always be the same in that the healer treats by touching or laying hands on – or just above – the body and channelling energy for the benefit of the horse at whatever level it needs it.

Although there are not that many qualified animal healers at present, this situation is set to change. The UK's largest healing organisation, the National Federation of Spiritual Healers (NFSH), recognises the need for a register of qualified animal healers and I am delighted to be consulting with them on how this should be done, including arrangements for specialised training which will qualify healers to join the referral register. In particular, there will need to be a special course for equine healers, which will be a major step forward to the benefit of horses and their owners.

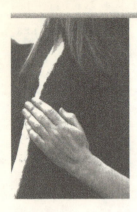

Conclusion

I HOPE that you have enjoyed this book and found some inspiration, some added insight into horses. I conclude by mentioning what we gain by giving hands-on healing to horses – that is, by doing so we learn deeper responsibility for horses in our care and also we gain knowledge of communicating on a higher level.

Giving the horse healing allows us the opportunity to gain a depth of knowledge we have probably not realised is possible. Through giving healing we are both learning and being taught at the same time as part of our spiritual evolution. You may wish to take your exploration and development of hands-on healing further and join a recognised organisation and I am sure that if you do will find it most fulfilling.

We are all part of the energy of this world and through healing can all share the positive experience of that energy. When you put your hands on your horse and offer it healing you will always be heard: by your horse, by the source of that healing energy and by your soul. It will do some good, on whatever level possible. And it will be good too for your own spiritual evolution.

I hope you will find that giving healing to your horse becomes a very rewarding and fundamental part of your life.

Margrit Coates

You and I

You are clever, you have power
You can make or you can break
You have marvellous potential?
You can choose the path you take

I have no such choice before me
I must live for the hour
I must walk the path of nature
I have feelings, but no power
You could banish world starvation
You could heal the sick and lame
But money's more desirable
And murders done for gain

I have no worldwide ambitions
I am happy just to live
I have naught for trade or barter
Only love, and that I give

Yet, I would live beside you
I would trust you, if I could
Though you abuse my friendship
And you often spilt my blood

But He, who sees each sparrow fall
And knows each stab of fear
And feels the silent agonies
Which no one else can hear,

Will intervene our destinies
Into His perfect plan
Though I am just an animal
And you, of course, are man

And when our souls stand face to face
On that advancing day
Which one will stand and shine
And which, for shame, will turn away?

You and I
by Tricia Sturgeon
Reproduced with
kind permission
from *Redwings in Poetry*

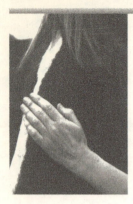

Useful addresses

Healing

The Margrit Coates Foundation for Animal Healing
PO Box No 1826
Salisbury
Wiltshire
SB5 2BH
UK
Website: www.thehorsehealer.com
Consultations, lectures and demonstrations. (A large stamped addressed envelope for details of the above appreciated.)

National Federation of Spiritual Healers (NFSH)
Tel: 01932 783164
E-mail: office@nfsh.org.uk
Website: www.nfsh.org.uk
Healer referral service. Details on courses and developing healing.

Practitioners in other complementary areas

British Holistic Veterinary Medicine Association (BHVMA)
Westgates
Muddles Green
Chiddingley
Lewes
Sussex
BN8 6HW
UK
Fax: 0113 2301106

American Holistic Veterinary Medical Association
2218 Old Emmorton Road
Bel Air
MD 21015
USA
Tel: 410-569-0795
Fax: 410-569-2346
E-mail: AHVMA@compuserve.com
Maintains a directory of members for referral information.

British Association of Homeopathic Veterinary Surgeons
Tel: 01367 718115
Website: www.BAHVS.com
Information on vets with an interest in homeopathy.

Association of British Veterinary Acupuncturists
85 Earls Court Road
London
W8 6EF
Tel: 0207 937 8215
Information about vets with an interest in acupuncture.

General Osteopathic Council
Osteopathy House
176 Tower Bridge Road
London SE1 3LU
UK
Tel: 020 7357 6655
For details on equine osteopaths.

USEFUL ADDRESSES

The Association of Chartered Physio-
therapists in Animal Therapy (ACPAT)
The Secretary
Morland House
Salters Lane
Winchester
Hampshire
SO22 5JP
UK
Tel: 01962 844390
Fax: 01962 863801
E-mail: acpat@clara.net
Website: www.acpat.org.uk
Supplies details of qualified equine physiotherapists.

Holistic Pets
Harestock Stud
Kennel Lane
Littleton, Nr Winchester
Hampshire
SO22 6PT
UK
Tel: 01962 885561
Fax: 01962 885567
E-mail: amanda@animaltherapy.co.uk
Website: www.animaltherapy.co.uk
Natural treatments for horses, dogs and cats. Homeopathy, physiotherapy, healing.

Top to Toe Days for Horses
Tel: 01962 885561
Fax: 01962 885567
Find out what your horse needs: natural remedies and therapies..

Rescue and rehabilitation centres for equines

Each of these organisations is in need of good homes and financial support.

World Horse Welfare
Anne Colvin House
Snetterton
Norfolk
NR16 2LR
UK
Tel: 01953 498682
E-mail: info@worldhorsewelfare.org
Website: www.worldhorsewelfare.org
Aims to protect horses from suffering and to alleviate suffering by world-wide rehabilitation and education programmes, and campaigns.

Redwings Horse Sanctuary
Hapton
Norwich
NR15 1SP
UK
Tel: 01508 481100
E-mail: info@redwings.co.uk
Website: www.redwings.co.uk
Provides sanctuary to horses, ponies and donkeys that are neglected, mistreated or homeless. Also works to relieve suffering through guidance and education of owners.

The Brooke
Tel: 020 7930 0210
E-mail: info@thebrooke.org
Website: www.thebrooke.org
Donations, subscriptions, legacies and fundraisers always much needed to help working equines, in the world's poorest communities, lead a comfortable life.

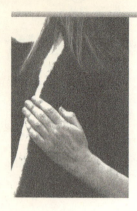

References and suggested further reading

Energy Medicine
James L. Oschman
Churchill Livingstone
ISBN 0 443 06261 7

Hands of Light
Barbara Ann Brennan
Bantam New Age Books
ISBN 0553345397

The Horse's Mind
Lucy Rees
Stanley Paul
ISBN 009 153660 X

How to Know God
Deepak Chopra
Rider Books
ISBN 0 7126 7035 1

Journey into Healing
Deepak Chopra
Rider Books
ISBN 0 7126 7068 8

The Nature of Horses
Stephen Budiansky
Pheonix Illustrated
ISBN 0 75380 531 6

Spiritual Healing
Liz Hodgkinson
Piatkus
ISBN 0 74991 007 0

Vital Energy
William Collinge
Thorsons
ISBN 0 00 710090 6

Working with your Chakras
Ruth White
Piatkus
ISBN 0 7499 1264 2

Author's acknowledgements

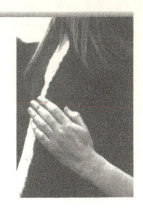

This book has been burning inside me for many years and I knew that it should be written for the benefit of horses – to take our understanding of them on to another level, a higher plane. For a long time it was not the right time, but something has changed with the dawning of the new millennium. Spiritual awareness for animals and humans is recognised as essential again. The horse's desperate, but vocally silent, plea to be helped was heard in the universe and then everything started to fall into place. Every time a horse looked at me and said 'help me' I worked harder to open the channels which would result in producing this book.

There are many people who I wish to thank, who have helped me in some way on my path and journey as a healer. All are healers in their own way, even if they haven't realised it yet, and there are too many to mention individually. They include my family and friends, colleagues and acquaintances, past and present.

However, I must thank my husband Peter without whose support, understanding and sacrifices I would not be free to follow my destiny.

Special thanks go to my partners at Holistic Pets, chartered animal physiotherapist Amanda Sutton who has been such an inspiration on my learning curve of gaining knowledge, and homeopathic vet Cheryl Sears, a truly holistic vet who understands the spiritual nature of animals and owners. I also acknowledge the help and guidance from the rest of our special and dedicated team – animal physiotherapists Jo Verhaeg, Esme Trevelayn and Claire-Maria Campbell.

I am also very grateful to equine vet Sue Devereux who found the time in her busy life to check relevant chapters of this book for technical accuracy.

I am indebted to Judith Kendra, Publishing Director of Rider Books, who gave me the opportunity to write this book, and then gave me the inspiration and advice I needed to be able to do it. Judith has been a guiding light in my foray as an author and has enabled me to bring the subject of hands-on healing for horses to a wide audience. It has been a joy as well to complete the book with project editor Sue Lascelles and copy editor Emma Callery.

Included in this book are the words to Kiki Dee's beautiful song 'Loving and Free' and I am so very grateful to Kiki for giving permission to reproduce this song, which she also wrote. I defy any equine lover to play this and not be incredibly moved, really tugged at the heart. Although the song wasn't written about horses you can see how relevant the words are to them, and how poignant.

Photographing horses is always difficult; the best pose is often the one when the photographer has left and gone home! I am very grateful therefore to Jon Banfield for successfully taking these photos for my book and to Mike and Nigel of Freelance Design for their help with illustrations.

Finally, I wish to thank all my clients, special people who love their horses so much that they have offered them the opportunity to have healing.

And the biggest thanks I give to the horses – noble, proud, intelligent, long suffering, misunderstood – who have taught me everything I know about hands-on healing for horses. One of those horses is featured on the front cover of this book – Michael, a 20-year-old pure-bred Arab – and I am grateful to him for his patience, kindness and good humour while the photographs were taken.

Margrit Coates

Index

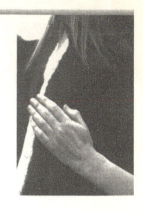

Abuse, of horses 49
Acupuncture, veterinary 17, 151, 152–3
  points 109
Affirmations 134
Aggressive handling 46
Alcohol, healing and 109
Alpha state 23
Anti-social behaviour 91–3
Apprehension 93–5
Arthritis 158
Atmosphere 60–1, 70–1
Attunement 2–3, 23–4, 33, 55
Auras 13, 31, 101, 112
'Awakened mind', the 23

Billington, Philip 5–6, 9
Biomagnetic fields 28
Blockages, emotional and memory 19, 26, 29, 31, 35
Box walking 80–1
Brachial major chakra 135–7
Brain wave patterns 23–4
Breathing problems 86–7
Brow chakra 139–40
Burr, Harold Saxon 61

Cade, Maxwell 23, 24
Case histories, healing 76–105
Chakras 20, 21, 48, 55, 72–3, 77, 109, 131–45, 147
Change, horses and 159
Coates, Peter 8
Colic 52
Communication
  horse's need for 53–5
  spiritual 46, 56–7, 108
Complementary therapies 8, 11–12, 71–2, 107, 150–5
Confinement 48–50
Cranial-sacral therapy 17, 144
Crown chakra 138
Crystals and gemstones, healing with 146–9

Daylight, insufficient 46–8
Death 29–30, 37–8, 96, 125

Dentistry 16, 17
Depression 48, 49, 51, 59, 75, 76–7
Destructiveness 78–9
Distant healing 32–3
Drugs, healing and 109

Early weaning 52, 54
Electricity pylons 59
Electromagnetic, energies 69, 131–45
  fields 21, 23–4, 26, 39, 115
  pulses 21
  therapy machines 26
Emotions, horses' 43–4, 56–7, 159
Endorphins 24, 74, 77, 81, 92, 100, 125
Energy
  balancing 17, 19, 67, 159
  and blockages 18–19, 28, 35, 50, 64, 75, 89, 102, 131
  and communication 56–7
  emotional 20, 40, 41, 64, 67, 69–71
  fields 18–19, 25–6, 28, 30–1, 61
  imbalances 19, 40, 41–2, 44, 55, 58
  lines 59
  medicine 2
  mental 20, 23–4
  negative 79, 84
  physical 20
  points 112
  shared 66–71, 79, 81, 88, 91
  spiritual 19
  transfers 18–24, 53, 54, 107
  and the universe 61–2
  weaknesses 64
  working with 106–7
Enkephalin 48
Environmental conditions 58–62
Epilepsy 87–8
Estabany, Oscar 27
Eyes, horses' 44–6

Geomagnetic fields 21, 59, 60
Geopathic conditions 58–60
Grad, Dr Bernard 26–7
Grief 49, 95–6, 96–7, 159

Hands, laying on of see Healing
Harfield, Gillian Makey 11, 12
Head collars, foals and 86
  fear of 89–91
Healers, registered 156–8
Healing
  and attunment 12, 71
  benefits of 25, 64
  case histories of 76–105
  and chakras 131–45
  children and 71–3
  and communication 55–6
  comfort of 24
  distant 32–3, 102–5, 127–8
  effectiveness of 25–8
  as first aid 121–2
  horses and people, differences in 65–9
  how to give 106–30
  and life force 18–19
  and lifestyle 128–9
  limitations of 125–7
  as preventative therapy 63–4
  reactions to 68, 118–20
  surrogate 90–1, 117
  and Top to Toe Days 16
  using crystals and gemstones 146–9
  what healers feel 123–4
  what horses feel 122, 123
Heart chakra 141–3
Help for horses 16–17
Herbal therapy 17, 151
Holistic Pets 16, 154
Holistic treatment 16–17, 107, 124, 150
Homeopathy 17, 151, 155
Homeostasis 19, 20, 63, 69, 124

167

Horses
    communication with 2–3
    and healing 20, 21–5, 62–3
    inner needs of 15, 20
    reasons for healing 39–41, 49, 124
    sensitivity of 31, 60–1, 61–2
    spirit of 29–30
    vulnerability of 12, 69, 110–11
Hunger 76

Illness, root causes of 63
Immune system, depressed 49, 53, 59, 64
Injuries 46, 159
Intent, importance of to healing 32, 37, 69, 115, 127–8, 134, 146
Intuitive healing 34–6, 108, 114

Journal of the Royal Society of Medicine 26

King, Mary 7
Kirlian photography 30
Krieger, Dolores 27

Life force 18, 29, 31
    and death 30, 38
Living matrix, the 31–2, 54
Loneliness 46, 125, 143
Love 33, 37, 110, 111, 141

Massage therapy 17, 154–5
Meditation 127, 129–30
Mental focus 23–4
Meridians 20, 21, 28, 48, 109, 152
Misunderstanding, between horse and human 42–3, 46

Mood changes 82–3
Murphy, Andrew 2

National Health Service (UK) 27, 71
Natural horsemanship 57, 92
Nutrition 51–2, 129

Osteopathy 17, 155
Over-stabling 49, 47–9, 51–2, 125

Pain 49
Photosensitisation reactions 48, 100
Physiotherapy 16, 17, 151, 153–4
Pluto 135
Post-viral syndrome 158

Rebalancing, of energy 15, 17, 22
Rehabilitation, horses and 17
Religion, healing and 36–7
Rest, need for 50
Riding, classical 17
Roberts, Monty 57
Root chakra 145
Royal College of Veterinary Surgeons (UK) 27, 156

Sacral chakra 144–5
Sacred communication 13
SAD (Seasonal Affective Disorder) 47
Sarcoids 53
Schooling, impatient 46
Schumann Resonance, the 23–4
Sears, Cheryl 16
Self-mutilation 78–9
Serotonin 51

Sessions, healing
    essentials for 108
    when to avoid 109
Sharing energy 43, 54
Skin
    conditions 53
    and healing 31–2
Sluggishness 104–5
Solar Plexus chakra 143–4
Soul, horses' 29, 44–6
Spirit 29, 47, 56–7
States of mind, importance of for healing 27, 41, 70–1, 109
Stillbirth 95–6
Stockdale, Tim 7
Stress 41, 42, 46, 49, 51, 63, 69, 92, 99
Sutton, Amanda 12, 17

Tait, Blyth 6, 9
Teamwork, horse and rider 17
Terminal illness 125, 159
Throat chakra 140
Top to Toe Days 15–16
Toxins 64, 100
Trust, horses' lack of 55–7
Tumours 59, 101–2, 158

Universal source of healing, the 21, 22, 28, 29, 32, 37, 106
Unpredictability 84–5

Verhaeg, Jo 82
Voice, horse's 1

Water, horses' need for 51–2
    and geophysical rhythms 59–60
Weather, changes to 52, 61–2
Weight loss 88–9
Wetzler, Gail 11
Work, and the horse's capability 41, 46, 57